TOWARDS TOTAL HEALTH

TOWARDS TOTAL HEALTH
A realistic approach to better living

Al Murray & Mike Bettsworth

B.T. BATSFORD LTD, LONDON

ACKNOWLEDGMENTS

We would like to extend out thanks to P.G.F. Nixon, MB, FRCP, Consultant Cardiologist at Charing Cross Hospital, for his assistance in cardiological matters, and for permission to reproduce his article 'We All Need Homeostasis'. To M.E. Carruthers, MD, MRC Path., MRCGP, Director of Clinical Laboratories, Maudsley and Bethlem Royal Hospitals, for his assistance in biochemical matters. To Mario Szewiel, ND, DO, MBNOA, Lecturer in Nutrition at the British College of Naturopathy and Osteopathy, for his contribution on diet and nutrition. To Jungeling Ltd for the weight training apparatus. To George Kirkley for the photography and to Bill Brandon and Grundy Engineering for the drawings and charts. Lastly, to F. Shipman, Dip. PE, City Gym Manager and to D. Valentine, Cert. Ed. (PE), City Gym Assistant Manager, for kindly posing in the exercises.

First published 1981
© Al Murray and Mike Bettsworth 1981

ISBN 0 7134 3413 9

Printed in Great Britain by
The Anchor Press Ltd
Tiptree, Essex
for the publishers B.T. Batsford Ltd,
4 Fitzhardinge Street, London W1H 0AH

Contents

Foreword

The vital importance of preventive health care is now recognized in virtually all Western countries. People are becoming increasingly aware of the limits of purely curative medicine. Most realize that many of the main factors governing their health are a question of a sensible lifestyle, a matter within their own control. Among men, for example, by far the greatest single cause of death over the age of 35 is coronary heart disease; and of its contributory causes, the most obviously preventable are smoking, obesity, inactivity and stress.

A guide such as this offers a basic explanation of these risks, and a commonsense way of avoiding them, often with a choice of techniques to suit individual people. The work of the City Gymnasium is a good example of how easily physical fitness can be brought within the reach of people leading busy lives, and this book complements that work in a very positive way.

Mrs Lynda Chalker, MP
Sir George Young, MP

*Joint Parliamentary Under-Secretaries of State
Department of Health and Social Security*

Introduction

The last few years have seen a steady increase in the number of books written on the subject of health, physical fitness, diet and stress. There have been many campaigns conducted by various sections of the media, by The Health Education Council and The Sports Council, all designed to make us more aware of the dangers inherent in unhealthy life-styles. We live in an age which acknowledges that heart disease, brought on by a number of allied factors, is the number one killer in the Western world; we live in an age which is learning more and more about the prevention and rehabilitation of cardiac disorders; we live in an age of increased leisure and one in which we are urged to partici-pate in a growing number of sports and physical pastimes. Yet despite this acute awareness and this growing volume of knowledge, we persist in inflict-ing upon ourselves a way of living which will lead to our early demise. And we collaborate with this situation in either of two ways. Either we ignore the deleterious effect which we *know* results from our, say, bad dietary habits or inactivity, or, and this is increasingly common, we decide to take action to improve our physical state, and embark on a regime of exercise or diet which is going to be actually harmful in its effect. That is, we take remedial steps without any advice.

It is for both these reasons that this book has been written. The information contained here is based upon the most up-to-date research available. Most of the research has been carried out at the City Gymnasium and Health Clinic in London. The exercise part of the programme has been developed by Alistair Murray, and is known as The Murray Work Loading System. Over 2000 cardiac patients have been successfully treated by the methods outlined in this book and many hundreds more are regularly taking advantage of the benefits offered at the City Gym. But how did it all begin?

Over twenty years ago, when Al Murray was a National Coach, he become increasingly alarmed at the intensity of exercise that was being given to unfit adults. He visited many commercial and other gymnasiums in this country and abroad, and every-where found that former athletes or training instruc-tors were setting up gymnasia and offering an exer-cise programme to unfit adults which was based on the training schedules of competitive athletes. In the case of fit young rugby players, for example, these gymnasia were, and still are, fulfilling a vital physical and community role. However, the rate of work being given to the older and more unfit adult was taking his pulse rate up to dangerously high levels. Nobody was to blame for this because there was nowhere in the country where training could be given to instructors to cater for the really unfit adult. The instructors had all been trained and were accustomed to deal with very fit, and usually very young people. In their enthusiasm they assumed that what was good for a school leaver suited a man or woman in his/ her forties or fifties. As a result of all this Al Murray decided to collect as much data as possible about pulse rates. He was working in his previous gym-nasium opposite St Paul's Cathedral, which he leased from The City of London Corporation. At this time, more than sixteen years ago, he was conducting tests with the late Dr Harold Lewis, then a Senior Physiologist with the Medical Research Council, to find out what physical qualities were best suited to particular physical activities. During this period Dr Lewis went to the United States of America and returned with a strong desire to conduct research into exercise as a means of heart disease rehabilita-tion; it was decided that he would use the Murray Gymnasium.

Unfortunately the gymnasium had been gutted by fire. This fact, and Dr Lewis's determination to continue the research with Al Murray, was to change the course of many lives. It was decided to abandon the previous work and to devote all effort towards work on cardiac rehabilitation and cardiac disease prevention. The gymnasium was rebuilt within nine months and research started. But because the leases were short-term ones, for the next eight or nine years the researchers were never certain that they would be able to carry out their work over long periods of time. A saviour came in the form of British Petroleum. This company had been sending executives to the Murray Gymnasium, and after two or three years, offered an alternative site in the base-

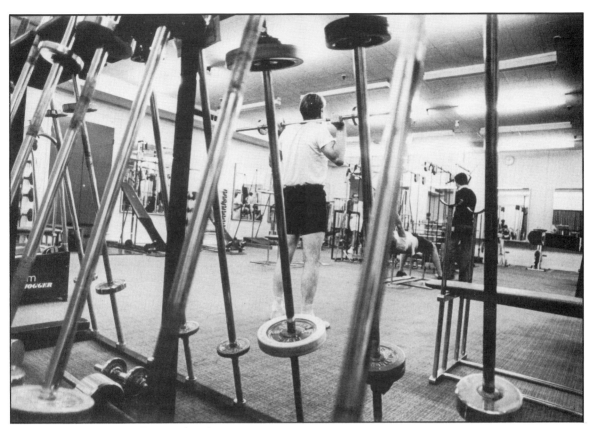

1 The City Gym clinic and research unit

ment of their headquarters, Britannic House. In June 1980 the Murray Gymnasium and Health Clinic celebrated six years' occupation there. And it was to be a gymnasium with a difference. Gone was the concern for competitive athletes and the research work that was being done on their behalf. The new gymnasium was designed so that it would function not only as a place where men and women could take regular supervised exercise, but also as a centre for the research work on cardiac prevention and rehabilitation which Dr Lewis so determinedly wished to carry out. Al Murray was selected to direct the exercise part of the programme because he was the only practising physical educator with the necessary knowledge and training to assist and pioneer this vital work. Even to this day the City Gym is the only place where instructors can be trained to administer exercise programmes to the really unfit adult, and it is still the only gymnasium which specializes in this work.

The early days were difficult, for despite the conviction of Dr Lewis and Mr Murray that a system of exercise based upon pulse rate control and other factors was the only sensible way to exercise the really unfit adult, and despite the obvious fact that other gymnasia were not designed to function in this specialized field for the reasons stated above, there was no financial help to offset research costs. The general public was unconvinced of the need for such research twenty years ago; the picture is so very different now. The small staff of Al Murray and Margarethe Holfeld, who is now a Director of the City Gym, soldiered on nonetheless.

As time passed and the work was beginning to be recognized, outside help was forthcoming. The then Minister for Sport, Denis Howell, and the Director of the Central Council for Physical Recreation (CCPR) at the time, Sir Walter Winterbottom, supported the research with a six-year financial grant from the Sports Council which was to be used for training physical education teachers. By this time the medical profession entered the scene. Professor Richard Edwards, now Professor of Metabolic Medicine at University College Hospital, London, helped the project, and after the untimely death of Dr Harold Lewis, Dr Peter Nixon, Consultant Cardiologist to the Charing Cross Group of Hospitals, and Dr Malcolm Carruthers, then Senior Lecturer

9

in the Department of Chemical Pathology at St Mary's Hospital Medical School, London, led the research work.

As time went on, the business world became convinced that the sort of programme offered at the City Gym was a good investment for them; healthy executives, they argued, were an important, though indirect, capital asset. Not only British Petroleum, but Burmah Oil, Grundy Engineering, even The Houses of Parliament and Champneys Health Resort, use Al Murray as a consultant. And there are many other concerns too.

The result of this research is that now the medical profession is convinced that post-cardiac patients can benefit from a controlled exercise programme. But, more important than this alone, side by side with the developments in exercise as a therapy, other factors have emerged as well. The situation now is that if the knowledge which we have were to be practised by the nation as a whole, there would be a significant increase in the health of our people, there would be a substantial reduction in the number of beds occupied in National Health hospitals, and, hence, a commensurate reduction in the cost of the National Health Service, and a massive reduction in the number of working days lost through illness of one sort or another. We are offering, in this book, a four-fold attack against ill-health, particularly against cardiac and its associated diseases.

And it is because much of what is contained here has never before appeared in print that this book is different from all others. The Murray Work Loading System has been a closely kept secret. The City Gym's system of treatment is unique, and it is only in the City Gym that work on exercise for heart disease is being carried out in depth. It is our eventual hope that instructors will come from within the National Health Service to be trained in our work. We further hope that the physical education profession as a whole will consider devising courses for training specialists to deal with the booming leisure industry, and to include in this training information about the physical needs of the really unfit adult. At the moment the profession is orientated towards the child and the young adult. But let it never be forgotten that the early signs which forebode cardiac disease are seen in quite young children; the symptom of hardening arteries is seen not only in the battle-weary middle-aged executive. Indeed, the problem of heart disease starts very young in the Westerner. Our hope is that due heed to what we have written will be paid by parents on behalf of their children, as much as by parents on behalf of themselves.

We aim to fill the gap between books on exercise for the young and fit, and books which deal solely with post-cardiac disease treatment. Further, we offer a total system of protection; many books identify one area of risk and concentrate only on that area. As opposed to them, we are offering a 'package deal', which deals with both health and fitness. We define health as the absence of disease and fitness as the ability to cope efficiently with physical and emotional problems.

We identify four main areas of risk. These are *smoking, obesity, inactivity* and *psychological stress.* Each of these factors, and they are often inter-related, will be discussed at length in the following chapters. They are the cause not only of heart disease, but of a whole range of other ailments, including ulcers, diabetes, respiratory and circulatory disorders, back and joint pains and migraines. Thus, if you take our advice, it can be truly said that training for what we are going to call protective physical fitness, as opposed to competitive physical fitness, is not only training for cardiac disease prevention, but also for that of many other ailments.

There is no way in which these risk factors can be either treated or detected in the average commercial gymnasium. The methods outlined in the following chapters show how every individual can adapt his remedial action to suit his exact needs. Age, sex, height, weight and medical history are all taken into account in deciding what is the correct amount of exercise, for example, any individual needs to be able to measure improvement in performance. Thus pulse control is an important feature of the training because the City Gym was the first place to discover the minimal work that needs to be done to produce measurable results. Much is made of stress, so, too, do we say something about the dangers of heavy smoking, and suggest how you can give up the habit. And we offer a chapter on diet which is straightforward and will not recommend eating habits beyond the pocket of the average individual.

In short, we do offer a 'package deal'. We are not merely concerned with physical exercise. Indeed, there are times when we recommend that exercise is really harmful. We are concerned with a definable individual — the really unfit adult — whom we define as a person who has a clinical condition which makes him or her a high risk as far as heart disease is concerned. We have calculated that 11-17 per cent of the subjects we have studied have such a condition, and are unaware of it. Such conditions include high blood pressure, high levels of cholesterol and free fatty acids in the blood; individuals who live under severe stress, suffer from insomnia, excessive tiredness and so on. And even the super-fit athlete can become a really unfit adult — and by the the age of thirty!

Our objective, then, is to allow individuals to recognize what they are doing to themselves by ignoring the effects of these four risk factors, and to give guidance on the prevention of cardiac disease by suggesting how these risks can be reduced. There is a complete chapter, at least, on each of those risk factors. We keep technical terms down to a minimum, and offer a diagnosis and system of treatment for each factor.

1 Stress-its causes and symptoms

Towards a definition

We have said that our aim in this book is to offer a package deal which, if taken *in toto,* will reduce the risk of heart disease, or if you have suffered cardiac malfunction, will help you to recover. We are concentrating on four main areas of risk. As a start let us consider the psychological factor of stress or excessive mental arousal. Arguably this is the most contentious factor as there are almost as many theories about the physiological mal-effects of stress as there are medical researchers. We will attempt to summarize the most important modern findings, and then suggest ways in which you can reduce the level of stress in your own life.

Much of the material available for study is highly technical and requires a knowledge of the biochemistry of the human body for it to be fully understood. Our aim is to be intelligible to the general reader and we have simplified this difficult material. In so doing we may not have satisfied the specialist reader; we make no apology for this, as the specialist reader will be able to fill in the gaps for himself.

As mentioned above, there are many theories about how stress, which is really distress, adversely affects the body's ability to function efficiently. Not all researchers in the field agree with all the theories. For our purpose, though, we can categorically state that stress is a major factor in producing heart disease. Of this no one in the medical profession now doubts. Below we suggest some of the ways in which stress affects our heart. In the following chapter we suggest ways in which you can reduce the incidence of stress.

What is stress? There are many definitions, and here are a few:

- Stress causes distress.

- Stress is the physiological response of the body to any demand made upon it.

- Stress is caused by environmental demands which require behavioural adjustment.

And there are many others. The one thing they have in common is that they imply that a stressful situation in some way arouses the body's organism to respond. This will be easily understood by everybody. If we go on a job interview or are going to ask a girl out for the first time we experience an increased heart rate, we may sweat and feel faint. We are under a degree of stress. Equally our heart rate is increased by kissing our beloved, just as much as it is increased by our suspecting there is a burglar in the house whom we must confront. Hence, by our definition which says that stress is the 'physiological response of the body to any demands made upon it', we may see that the cause of stress, the stressor, may be equally pleasant or unpleasant. We may now understand what Hans Selye, one of the father figures of stress research, means when he says that stress is the non-specific response of the body to any demand made upon it.

Before going further we ought to say that not all stress is harmful. We have all experienced the exhilaration of buoying ourselves up to key pitch in order to achieve an important goal. It may be the feeling we experience before an important race, or the challenge of overcoming an academic hurdle, or the flowing of adrenaline just before we propose to the person we love. This kind of heightened awareness is important to our physical and mental well-being. However, we know that if we were to live our every minute at such a pitch we would soon become 'drained'. A certain amount of mental arousal is good for us. Continual pressure of this sort will wear us down.

Over forty years ago Dr Selye coined an expression of the triphasic nature of the body's response to stress. He called it the 'general adaptation syndrome' (GAS), and identified three stages in the body's reaction to stress:

Stage 1 The alarm reaction

Once the body has perceived a stressor it brings its defence mechanism into play. The brain activates the pituitary gland which discharges the adreno-corticotrophic (ACTH) hormone into the blood. ACTH causes the adrenal glands to secrete corticoids such as adrenalin. At the same time the production of sugar as a ready source of energy is increased. We will ignore the many other chemical changes; suffice it to say that the body is put on full alert to deal with the emergency.

Stage 2 The resistance stage
While the body can cope adequately with the stressor it continues to resist. It seeks to maintain a state of homeostasis (or balance), by adapting to the stressor.

Stage 3 The exhaustion stage
However, the body's adaptive resources are finite. The acquired adaptation is replaced by the initial alarm reaction. The body becomes unable to cope with the situation, increased wear and tear is experienced, and the individual may die.

What we have just said about GAS has been said in another way by Dr Peter Nixon, Consultant Cardiologist at Charing Cross Hospital. We think it useful, before going further, to quote his article ('We All Need Homeostatis') in full.

The householder uses a thermostat to help maintain the constancy of the hot water system. The body likewise uses a variety of homeostatic devices to protect the constancy of the internal milieu against the changes which might be caused by our variable responses to the ever-changing circumstances in which we live. Thirst protects against

dehydration, for example, and goose-pimples help to defend us from hypothermia. Fatigue warns us against carrying on until we are exhausted, but the programmes and duties of our lives make us deaf to its voice and conditioning makes us scorn to listen out for it.

The Human Function Curve [see fig 1] is a paradigm illustrating the way we go 'over the hump' into exhaustion and deteriorating function if we allow ourselves to go on being aroused hard enough and long enough past the level of healthy fatigue. In exhaustion, our trying harder to overcome the deterioration just makes us less efficient because the extra effort increases the arousal, and our performance is already on a downslope. Fighting to close the gap between what we actually can do and what we think is intended of us only widens it. High levels of arousal interfere with the restorative value of sleep and so aggravate the exhaustion.

To be exhausted is to court danger from every point of view. There are no reserves of energy for coping with unexpected and unfamiliar stimuli, and it is difficult to adapt to change. We lose the ability to habituate, i.e. to enjoy the benefits of the decreasing arousal which is part of 'getting used to things' and 'settling down'; and to discriminate between the essential and inessential demands upon our energy. The consequent loss of self-esteem and rise of unpleasant tension generate more arousal. Aggression flares up, often inappropriately, and destroys the goodwill of potential allies. Maladaptive coping tactics flourish: particularly serious is the acceptance of serious sleep deprivation as 'normal'. Leadership comes to depend more upon age and seniority than ability, and defences are erected against

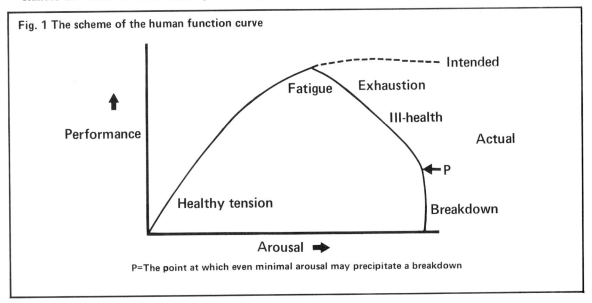

Fig. 1 The scheme of the human function curve

Performance ↑

Intended

Fatigue   Exhaustion

Ill-health

Actual

← P

Healthy tension   Breakdown

Arousal ➡

P=The point at which even minimal arousal may precipitate a breakdown

any change of routine which might call for initiative and energy. It becomes impossible to live and work with the chronically exhausted individual and social cohesion is disrupted. In the severest forms of exhaustion the individual bogs himself down in rage and despair: he cannot go on, he can't opt out, and everlasting discussion will never produce an acceptable compromise.

Exhaustion with rage and despair is particularly dangerous from the homeostasis point of view. The commonest immediate causes seem to be the loss of ability to understand and control our circumstances: people-poisoning; excessive time-pressures; and resentment about changes imposed by others in families and social organisations. The usual response is to deny the problems or to reject them; and to press on regardless, but ever downwards, in increasingly furious displacement activity. These vicious circles cannot be carried on indefinitely. Sooner or later homeostasis is violated, and malfunctions ultimately capable of causing a breakdown [at P in fig. 1] are set in train because the constancy of the internal milieu cannot be maintained. The phase after exhaustion on the downslope of the Curve is ill-health, and its nature depends upon the age and circumstances of the individual. The heart can become inefficient, uncomfortable or painful in action, and subject to various sorts of erratic and rapid beating. Angina pectoris, coronary insufficiency and myocardial infarction may be the cause of the breakdown when the demands of a highly aroused and exhausted individual outstrip the capacity of his coronary circulation. The blood pressure climbs or swings too high for too long in response to common or garden stimuli; the blood levels of cholesterol, triglycerides, sugar and uric acid tend to rise and the blood clots too readily. Fluid retention is common and resistance to infection is reduced. People become accident-prone. Disorders of the stomach, duodenum and bowel are common, and the breathing may be uncomfortable. Aches and pains from the limbs, joints, 'discs and backs' are the rule rather than the exception.

Some incredibly tough individuals can violate their homeostasis and produce ill-health for years on end before they run out of energy or break down. Many of them are addicted to a way of life which is self-destructive in the end because it violates homeostasis over and over again.

In medical practice the traditional and logical way to diagnose the forms of ill-health which come from being aroused far beyond the level of healthy fatigue is to remove the exhaustion and hyper-arousal, perhaps with a sleeping-resting regime of the sort used to rescue fighters from the over-exposure of battle conditions. When the ill-health disappears with the recovery of homeostasis the diagnosis has been confirmed and the first therapeutic step has been taken. The second step is education: the individual who wishes to control his own health learns not to jeopardise his freedom by violating his homeostasis, and then trains himself to become fit enough and skilful enough to go forward as a health 'winner' where previously he was a 'loser'.

Unfortunately, we have been passing through an era in medicine in which logic and common-sense have sometimes been replaced by the pharmaceutists' propaganda which urges little more than the removal of symptoms with drugs. However, it does not take much to see, for example, that bringing down the blood pressure with a drug is not the same as removing exhaustion and the smell of defeat. Inhibiting the heart's responses with a betablocker such as propanolol is not the same as dealing with frustration, exhaustion and despair. The heart is an interesting organ: it hasn't a telephone line to tell consciousness when it has been used badly for too long, and it tends to complain with pain when it has been ill-used to a dangerous degree. I am glad to say that the ability to silence this voice with drugs and operations is not yet universally accepted as a high point of medical progress.

It should be clear from what I have written that well-trained counsellors have an extraordinarily large wasteland to develop. It includes teaching children to recognise and deal with the consequences of hyperarousal and exhaustion, and teaching adults how to become health 'winners' instead of 'losers'. Self-awareness can be enhanced. Homeostasis violators can be recognised, helped to transcend their unfortunate circumstances and responses, and eased out of their addiction. The social, managerial and therapeutic skills in our communities can be increased. People who have gone down into ill-health or breakdown can be helped to get well or to make the best of their infirmity. The more the health professionals give impersonal treatments, and select and organise themselves to have neither the taste nor the time for personal commitment, the greater will be the field for the counsellor. In my opinion, more than half the people carrying the labels of hypertension and coronary disease could achieve healthy functiom if they learned how to be rid of hyperarousal, exhaustion and sleep-deprivation. A great advance would be made if they were taught nothing more than to be still sometimes, and to cultivate a healthy respect for fatigue.

Thus writes Dr Nixon. We have quoted his article in full because it serves as a useful starting point for our discussion. Much that he writes is beyond the immediate scope of this book, but what he says should give everyone food for thought. In what follows it is our aim to expand upon much that he has said. But by now you will see that there is little essential difference between what Selye calls the 'general adaptation syndrome' and what Nixon calls the 'human function curve'.

Nixon has mentioned that there is a number of stress-related diseases. It may be useful at this point to list a few of the commonest.

Stress-related diseases and symptoms

Hypertension — high blood pressure
Coronary disease
Allergies
Migraine and tension headaches
Lowering of immunity to infection
Ulcers
Insomnia
Indigestion
Diarrhoea
Constipation
Excessive drinking or smoking
Diabetes

This list is mentioned early on in the discussion as it should be made clear that stress is not a rare condition experienced only by the work-hungry business executive. All of us at one time or another experience distressing stress, and we should be aware of this as much as we should be aware of the advantages of a good diet and of regular exercise.

Some years ago two American doctors produced a table of what they called Life Change Units, and accorded a certain numerical score to a variety of events. Instead of counting calories we are invited to count Life Change Units. The higher our total of these units, the more are we likely to suffer from serious physical or psychological illness. We reproduce the list below. To calculate your own score, go through the list and tick the life changes that have occurred to you during the last year. Add up the total number of points. As a guide to assessing your own level of risk one can say:

150-199 life change units give you a mild chance of becoming ill in the next year.
200-299 and you are moderately at risk.
Over 300 life change units and you are in a group very likely to suffer from serious illness.

Events	Life change units
Death of a spouse	100
Marital separation	65
Death of close family member	63
Personal injury or illness	53
Marriage	50
Loss of job	47
Marital reconciliation	45
Retirement	45
Change in health of family member	44
Wife's pregnancy	40
Sex difficulties	39
Gain of a new family member	39
Change in financial status	38
Death of a close friend	37
Change to a different kind of work	36
Increase or decrease in arguments with spouse	35
Taking out a large home mortgage	31
Foreclosure of mortgage or loan	30
Change in work responsibilities	29
Son or daughter leaving home	29
Trouble with in-laws	29
Outstanding personal achievement	28
Wife beginning or stopping work	26
Revision of personal habits	24
Trouble with business superior	23
Change of work hours or conditions	20
Change in residence	20
Change in schools	20
Change in recreation	19
Change in social activities	18
Taking out a small home mortgage	17
Change in sleeping habits	16
Change in number of family get-togethers	15
Change in eating habits	15
Vacation	13
Minor violation of law	11

The above table was drawn up by Dr Thomas Holmes and Dr Richard Rahe, of the University of Washington School of Medicine. Many case histories were studied, and although the table, like so much research, is retrospective rather than prospective, it is easy to see that the common events contained in it do affect our lifestyles. Subsequent comparison by Holmes and Rahe on over 5000 individuals show that there is a high correlation between their life change scores and subsequent medical history.

It is hoped that by now you realize that many of the minor ailments which we come to tolerate after a while may be symptoms of what is essentially an 'invisible' disease — distress. Further it will be seen that the common incidents of most of our lives are probably the partial cause of the ailments. Hence you will see why it has been said that it is not the jet-travelling executive alone who is at risk. Indeed, the highest incidence of cardiac disease in Great Britain is centred in the south-west of Scotland where there is much unemployment and poverty.

Stress has sometimes been called the 'new disease', and its effects the 'hidden epidemic'. There is little in the literature of past cultures which speaks of stress or nervous breakdown. However, there is much in more recent literature which hints that a tranquil way of life is good for our souls. Modern research indicates that the sort of philosophy which does our souls good is equally good for our bodies. It is, in fact, only within the last forty or fifty years that scientists have been able to attach physiological explanations of psychological conditions, but the same response, whether we call it the 'general adaptation syndrome' or, as is better known the 'fight-or-flight' response, has been long known.

The fight-or-flight response

The American physiologist Walter Cannon was the first to coin the phrase 'fight-or-flight'. He used it to describe the responses available by the body to meet any emergency. It is possible that we have inherited these responses from our cavemen ancestors who, when faced with a sabre-toothed tiger, had the choice of running from it or fighting it. We see the same reaction in an angry dog. If it is going to fight, it snarls and its hackles raise. If it is going to flee, it does so with its tail between its legs. On the cellular level, if a poison enters the body it is either chemically destroyed or it is secreted by the body. From our own experience, say when a row is brewing with a colleague or spouse, we either have a row or we become conciliatory. In all cases the response by the body to the threat is easy to state, for the response is automatically controlled by the autonomic nervous system. Sometimes the word 'autonomic' is replaced by either 'involuntary' or 'sympathetic'.

When we are reacting to a 'fight-or-flight' situation, the following physiological changes occur:

— muscles tense
— the breathing rate increases
— stored sugar and body fats are released into the bloodstream
— the pupils of the eyes dilate
— red blood cells pour into the bloodstream carrying more oxygen to the muscles
— blood-clotting mechanics are activiated to deal with any injury
— heart rate and blood pressure rise rapidly
— digestion ceases so that blood may be carried to the muscles and brain
— sweating and salivation increase
— the pituitary gland causes the endocrine gland to release extra hormones
— bowel and bladder muscles loosen
— adrenalin, epinephrin and norepinephrin pour into the bloodstream
— our whole sense of 'awareness' is heightened

But we are not cavemen. Because we are rational beings, any eliciting of the fight-or-flight response nowadays tends to be of little use. If we have a row with the boss we can neither punch him on the jaw nor run away from him. We perceive the stressor and have to adjust our behaviour accordingly. Sustained evocation of the alarm reactions listed above may ultimately lead to our death through heart attack.

There are, of course, rare instances, perhaps in war, when the basic reaction must be necessary. But so often individuals turn on the reaction irrelevantly, such that the body may be in a permanent state of readiness or tension. If we are lucky the only effect of this prolonged tension will be that we are known as people who 'burn up a lot of nervous energy' or who 'find it difficult to relax'. At worst the saturation of the body with the 'emergency hormones' will result in damage to the vital organs or the nervous system, which will result in serious illness or death. Let us look a little more closely at the anatomy and physiology of stress before going on to look at how stress can bring about various physical disorders.

The anatomy and physiology of fight-or-flight

As already mentioned, when the fight-or-flight response is evoked, the area of the brain known as the hypothalamus is electrically stimulated to bring into play the automatic nervous system. The hypothalamus stimulates the pituitary gland to produce ACTH which enters the bloodstream. The ACTH reaches the adrenal glands which are situated above the kidneys. The adrenals are endocrine glands consisting of two parts. The inner core, or medulla, secretes adrenaline and related hormones, and the outer layer, or cortex, produces hormones, sometimes known as corticoids, such as cortisone. It is the release of all these hormones which causes all the signs of a body under stress — heavier breathing, increase in blood pressure, release of fats etc. All the changes associated with fight-or-flight are reflex and wonderfully integrated. However, it is possible to stimulate the response artificially, and experiments done on rats show that prolonged evocation of the response has very harmful effects.

The rats were injected with toxic substances, for example, or placed under some other form of stress and the reaction on their adrenal glands, thymus and lymph nodes measured. The adrenal glands became discoloured and enlarged because of the deposits of fatty tissue as a result of the increased metabolic activity the stress evoked. The thymus, a lymphatic organ situated in the chest, and the lymph nodes, whose function it is mainly to attack foreign bodies in the system, atrophied (became smaller). And, indeed, there were signs that the alarmed rats developed stomach ulcers.

There is no reason to suppose that the same effects will not occur in the human body if it is aroused too highly and for too long. There is one school of thought which even suggests that the amount of resources the body has available for dealing with emergencies is limited and that it is possible to use up the 'emergency supplies'. Not everyone agrees with this, but the evidence from the rat experiments would suggest that if we do not use up our resources, at least we may reduce or adversely affect the quality of the stress.

It is now time to look at the relationship between stress and physical disorders.

Stress and coronary disease

a. Atherosclerosis (arteriosclerosis)

Atherosclerosis is an unnatural narrowing of the arteries caused by the deposition of fatty globules on the inside walls of the arteries. While it is true that blood clots and calcium will also be deposited in the lumen of the artery (i.e. in the hollow part through which the blood flows), it would appear that the main cause of atherosclerosis is the level of blood fats. The two most significant fats are cholesterol and triglyceride. It seems that sudden stress raises the level of triglycerides in the body, and that prolonged stress results in an increase in serum cholesterol. Research on racing car drivers has revealed that before and during a race their triglyceride levels were up. Tax specialists were found to have elevated serum cholesterol levels as they approached the end of the accounting year. As well as raising blood fat levels, stress may also increase the tendency of the blood to clot. These clots may be deposited on the artery walls.

b. Hypertension (high blood pressure)

High blood pressure has rightly been called the hidden epidemic. Its symptoms are by and large invisible, but it is the direct cause of most deaths in the Western world. Blood pressure is the propelling force within the blood vessels which causes the various nutrients to be carried round the body. A higher than normal blood pressure is one of the causes of atherosclerosis.

Just as stress increases the levels of blood fats, so too does blood pressure rise during periods of stress. These two reactions become compounded.

The increased blood pressure forces more cholesterol into the artery wall. With an increase in blood pressure the heart has to work harder to force the blood around the body. The result of this is that the heart increases in size. This enlargement means that it requires more blood to flow through its own arteries so that it can cope with its own increased demands. If it does not receive sufficient nutrients then the muscle tissue will die. The heart will not receive the nutrients it requires because the coronary arteries will not be able to enlarge sufficiently and because atherosclerosis is developing within these arteries. Thus a vicious circle is developing.

c. Stroke

A further consequence of high blood pressure and atherosclerosis is that blood vessels have a tendency to burst. If this occurs in the brain then a brain haemorrhage is the result. If arteries leading to the brain become blocked, a stroke is the result, because the brain is not being supplied with oxygen and the necessary nutrients. If the brain cells are thus starved they die, and their function ceases. The effects of a stroke can be mild or very severe, permanent or temporary, but it is not uncommon for stroke victims to lose their speech, become paralysed and, in extreme cases, to die.

d. Hypertension and the kidneys

The kidneys function in the maintenance of blood pressure control. If blood pressure drops the kidneys release hormones that increase blood pressure. If the vessels within the kidney becomes even mildly atherosclerotic then obviously the amount of blood flowing to the kidneys will be reduced, and the kidneys will shrink. Further than this, blood pressure within the kidney will become lower. As a result the kidney responds by releasing more hormones and this increases the blood pressure throughout the whole body. Therefore the likelihood of developing further atherosclerosis occurs, and the same vicious cycle is being repeated.

Thus hypertension adversely affects the heart, the brain and the kidneys. And we know that stress causes an increase in blood pressure.

e. Angina pectoris

Angina pectoris occurs when an area of the heart is deprived of blood. The sufferer feels a tightness in the chest and pain may travel down the arm or up to the neck and jawbone. This condition can be brought on by emotional tension.

f. Heart attack

From all that we have said in this section it will readily be seen that if the coronary arteries become blocked, either through atherosclerosis or by a thrombus (clot) which has formed elsewhere being lodged in them, then the portion of the heart served by these arteries will be starved of blood. The result will be coronary insufficiency. The resultant lack of oxygen will cause myocardial infarction (heart attack).

Stress and ulcers

In the experiments on rats mentioned before it was said that one result of applying 'pressure' to the rats was the development of stomach ulcers. It is now believed that stress is a major cause of peptic ulcers. These ulcers form when the digestive juices burn a hole in the lining of the stomach and more particularly, the duodenum. It is the case that in times of high emotional stress the digestive enzymes and hydrochloric acid are secreted. This is particularly the case if the stressor is not known in advance and the body has no time to anticipate the change in circumstances.

It is possible, too, that cigarette smoking, alcohol and even the release of cortisone may lead to stomach ulcers. And certainly it has been shown experimentally that cortisone excesses are associated with times of nervous tension.

Stress and diabetes

Diabetes is caused by an insulin insufficiency which results in an inability of diabetics to absorb sufficient blood sugar into their cells. The pancreatic hormone insulin has the function of metabolizing glucose. When the glucose is not broken down it accumulates in the body causing severe chemical imbalance. The body is deprived of fuel and, hence, has to burn up its stores of fat.

Stress, which increases blood sugar levels, has an adverse effect on diabetics, in that they may be forced to secrete insulin excessively to cope with the blood sugar, with the result that the pancreas may become weakened, and the individual suffer from acute insulin deficiency. Stress has therefore been implicated in being a cause of diabetes.

Stress and immunity to infection

The human body is constantly being attacked by 'bugs'. We are subjected to assaults by microscopic organisms which are foreign to our system and which, if we are unable to combat them, will cause us to become ill and may even kill us. The body has two primary ways to combat these invaders: inflammation and specific immunity. When dangerous microbes enter the body the tissue around them swells and surrounds them, thus preventing their entering the bloodstream and causing damage. Often these isolated organisms can be killed by white blood cells.

When the foreign invaders manage to survive this inflammatory isolation the body must then attack them using antibodies. The microbes eventually come across the antibodies which attach themselves to them, thus causing a barrier between the invader and nutrients. The microbe is thus starved to death. The system works because the antibody and the microbe have compatible shapes and electrical charges. Once the invader has been recognized the body manufactures large quantities of the compatible antibody.

Under emotional stress the portion of the brain known as the hypothalamus causes the pituitary gland to release adrenal hormones called glucorticoid hormones. It is known that the presence, in excess, of these hormones makes our immunity system less efficient. The inflammatory response is less effective, and the body manufactures fewer antibodies. This is why we say of a person who is 'run-down', that his resistance is lowered. Thus the fight-or-flight response can be a direct cause of many maladies, particularly those caused by virus infection. It is even thought that some maladies, such as rheumatoid arthritis and colitis are attributed to stress.

The foregoing explanations will certainly support the theories of Drs Rahe and Holmes which, as explained, relate illness with changes in lifestyles and conditions.

Stress and headaches

It is often the case that very busy people suffer from headaches. These are people who find it difficult to relax, whose muscles are always tense even when they are not actively doing anything. The pain often affects the shoulders and neck before creeping into the head. These so-called tension headaches may well be attributable to stress.

The migraine headache, a much more painful condition, can be caused by a number of factors. Some postulate a dietary cause, others suggest heavy lifting as a cause, while others attribute the agony of migraines in women to the birth control pill. But it seems certain that stress is a major cause of migraines. The intense pain is caused by the dilation of blood vessels in the scalp. These vessels can become inflamed and it is possible that there are bio-chemical changes occurring simultaneously. It is a fact that few migraine sufferers undergo an attack when they, themselves, are in a stressful situation. It is when the pressure has been lifted that the attacks seem to occur. It seems possible, also, that migraine sufferers belong to the type of insecure person. And insecure persons suffer from stress.

Now that we are talking about types of personality, it seems appropriate to investigate more closely the relationship between 'stress' and 'type'. This brings us to Friedman and Rosenman.

Type personalities

About a quarter of a century ago two American heart specialists, Dr Meyer Friedman and Dr Ray Rosenman, conducted an investigation to see if there was any relationship between personality type and cardiac disease. They studied 35,000 men for a period of ten years, and came to the conclusion that there is a relationship between personality type and cardiac disease. It is only fair to say that not all cardiologists accept their findings, not least because the studies tended to be retrospective rather than prospective. In effect it is the case that, because the studies were retrospective, it may well have been that the personality was affected by the heart condition, rather than the heart condition being caused by the personality type. Be that as it may, there seems to be convincing evidence that some people are more prone to cardiac disease than others. Friedman and Rosenman identified Type A and Type B individuals.

Characteristics of Type A

Type A is the individual more likely to suffer from cardiac disease. He is always working against time, seeking to achieve more and more in less and less time. He tends to be aggressive and hostile, and though externally self-confident, may well be insecure underneath. Hence, he has to be continually proving himself, either by acquiring more money, or by achieving recognition through pulling off a *coup* of some kind. His lifestyle may be sedentary. He may smoke and drink too much and eat a rich diet.

Physiologically Type A has a chronically elevated blood serum level, and an excess of the stress hormones in his blood. His insulin level in the blood is similarly elevated and he takes three or four times longer to remove the food cholesterol ingested with each meal than other people. Type A is more likely to have blood clots forming in the coronary arteries than is Type B. This, together with the excess of insulin which is always associated with atherosclerosis, shows just how much at risk Type A is. We need hardly add that Type A is likely to suffer from hypertension.

Characteristics of Type B

Type B is the opposite. In the words of Friedman and Rosenman he is 'rarely harried by desires to obtain a wildly increasing number of things or participate in an endlessly growing series of events in an ever decreasing amount of time.' B is three times less likely to contract cardiac disease even if he is higher on other risk factors, such as smoking, than his aggressive opposite.

What to do

It would be a mistake to imagine that the overactive Type A can have his personality changed. It would be undesirable to try and change him anyway. However, Friedman and Rosenman do recommend that Type A characteristics, which are very harmful, can be eliminated. It is a question of rechannelling this energy and attitudes. For it is not only the business executive who suffers from stress; all of us who have to make behavioural adjustments because of environmental pressures are under stress.

The people in the Glasgow region of Scotland, for example, have a very high incidence of coronary disease which is stress-related. It is possible that they smoke and drink more heavily than normal, they seem to indulge in less physical activity, and the overcrowded, tenement life gives them acute environmental problems. It would be impossible to say that stress causes them to smoke and drink more, or that smoking and drinking causes their heart disease, and hence, their stress. The important point to be realized is that stress can be brought about by the opposite of the executive syndrome.

It would appear that the more we are at one with our environment the less are we likely to suffer from stress. One cardiologist has spoken of the need for a 'good support network'. He means by this a sense of belonging to one's immediate environment, being on good terms with one's family, and having an orderly and harmonious business life. It was the case in the United States, for example, among expatriate Japanese, that the incidence of heart disease was lower among the Japanese who maintained their traditional lifestyle in the new country, than among those who became Americanized. The second group seem to have been more susceptible to cardiac disease because their 'support network' was lacking.

In general terms, then, it can be said that if we are able to identify the areas in which we suffer from stress at home, work and in our immediate environment, we should be able to eliminate them. This is, of course, easy to say! On the next page is the advice which Friedman and Rosenman give to Type A personalities. You can modify their advice to suit your own situation — bearing in mind that the elimination of excessive stress is only one of our aims. If you modify your diet, smoking and exercise habits at the same time you are automatically reducing stress. If you reduce the incidence of mental arousal you may not be, say, a compulsive eater. More exercise will lessen your desire to smoke, and so on. All the time we are dealing with a kind of chicken and egg situation.

How Type A can modify his behaviour

Set Priorities — don't devote as much time to trivia as you do to the important things.

Revise your daily schedule — allow more time to complete various tasks. Do away with jobs that are likely to upset your over-all well-being. Learn to say no. Get up earlier in the morning so that you have time to think or go for a walk.

Examine yourself honestly — are you being too ambitious and unrealistic in your life goals? Are you spending too much time at work and not enough at play? Is your work being pursued so relentlessly that the spiritual side of your life is neglected?

Decide what your aim in life is — set yourself goals in work and in your private life. Write down your aims and review them often.

Conform — recognize the value of tradition and social ritual.

Work in peace — many people of Type A work in a chaotic milieu which accords with their sense of time urgency. Keep a tidy office. Put aesthetic objects in it. Learn not to talk all the time. Let others speak and listen to what they say.

Take a lunch break — and make it a break. Don't gobble down a sandwich while dictating to your secretary. Cut down on the number of business luncheons. Make the meal an occasion when you can forget your work for a time.

Don't procrastinate — Type A likes to work against the clock and to deadlines. Organize your time better so that you meet deadlines in comfort. By so doing you will be able to spend more time alone enjoying other pursuits.

Don't be aggressive — avoid people who bring out your hostility. If you meet them try treating them with good humour.

The above advice directly refers to Type A. It will be seen, though, that it is relevant to many of us who would not regard ourselves necessarily as Type A personalities. The following chapter suggests various relaxation techniques which will allow you to become a calmer and more satisfied person.

2 Relaxation techniques

We saw in the last chapter that psychological stress or excessive mental arousal can seriously affect our health. Suggestions were given for some of the causes of this arousal and it was seen that much of the trouble comes from our being unable to cope with such stress. 'Coping' is a key word as far as we are concerned, because a situation which causes stress to one person can be a neutral external incident to another. Therefore we can say that it is not so much that an external stimulus will cause us stress, as that it is how we react to that stimulus. Shakespeare, as always, hit the nail on the head when he wrote:

> There is nothing either good or bad,
> But thinking makes it so.

As the complexities and pace of life of the world increase, and they certainly do not seem to be getting simpler, it seems that the only way we can control our particular stressors is by the application of relaxation techniques within ourselves.

We have already said that the advice given to Type A personality is applicable to all of us. To come to terms with our family, job and environment generally, we may have to modify our aims, reset priorities and change our beliefs. These are changes which we can make with a will to succeed. However, in this chapter we wish to outline some of the major relaxation techniques which have been found to be helpful to all sorts of people, and which help us to increase our mental arsenal, the better to cope with stress.

The words 'meditation' and 'relaxation' will be used frequently, and it is worth stating from the outset that we are not allying any particular system of control technique to any religious or mystical experience. Equally, of course, we are not suggesting that a particular form of religious experience offered by a specific creed is unacceptable. This is merely a book about cardiac-disease prevention, and it is not concerned with a study of comparative religious belief! The following techniques are presented in no particular order. For all of them we claim that the negative physiological and psychological responses to external stimuli mentioned in the previous chapter are lessened. Thus stress is reduced, and the risk of heart disease lessened.

Meditation as an aid

Most of us know that a meditative experience requires the following four basic elements of:

- a quiet and peaceful environment
- an object to concentrate on
- a passive mental attitude
- a comfortable physical position

These same four prerequisites of meditation are recommended here as an aid to the exercise programme. It is suggested, and results would substantiate this, that when a person is engaged in, say, the weight-training programme, he will work better by concentrating all his thoughts on the work in hand. If one's train of thoughts veers away, one can guide it gently back. This will not only improve the way in which the exercises are being done, but, by emptying the head of the fragmentary thoughts which bombard us all, the mind, too, will be able to relax. And it does not matter that as soon as the exercise programme is over, the head becomes filled with heterogeneous ideas; during the 20-minute exercise period the mind was allowed to forget the problems of the external world.

The relaxation response

As if anticipating us, the relaxation response was formulated at Harvard's Thorndike Laboratory and at Boston's Beth Israel Hospital by Dr Herbert Benson. He has pointed out that there is nothing inherently new in his 'method'; he says that it is the amalgam of many oriental and occidental practices. He also suggests that whereas many of the meditative practices upon which he draws are rooted in religious and mystical experience, we can all benefit from them even when we do not subscribe to the dogma which originally surrounded them. We need the four elements listed above. That is:

A quiet, peaceful setting – a place where we can shut ourselves off from external distractions, and therefore avoid internal, fragmentary thought.

An object to concentrate on – this object may be a word or sound which we can repeat. It may be a symbol or it may be concentrating on a particular feeling. Whatever it is, we must evoke it when distracting thoughts enter our consciousness.

A passive mental attitude — and this Dr Benson says is the most important element. Such an attitude involves the emptying of the mind of all thoughts and responses, including that of worrying about intruding thoughts as they appear. In other words one must allow these random thoughts to enter the mind and then pass on.

A comfortable position — we have all experienced the unpleasant feeling of not being able to get comfortable. We cannot sleep if the bed is uncomfortable. We cannot concentrate on a play or a film if our sitting posture causes us ill ease. We need a position which we can adopt for 20 minutes. For the relaxation response a sitting posture is recommended — a lying down one may well lead to sleep, and as we are seeking to alter the consciousness of the individual, putting him unconscious will not help!

Once these four elements have been adopted the following steps should be taken.

1 Sit quietly in a comfortable position.
2 Close your eyes.
3 Relax all your muscles so that they feel heavy. Start at the toes, and work systematically through all the muscle groups ending with the scalp.
4 Breathe through the nose. As you exhale, slowly utter the word 'one' to yourself in a protracted exhalation. Your cycle should be, breathe *in* . . . *out*, 'one', *in* . . . *out*, 'one'.
5 Follow this procedure for 15 to 20 minutes. Open your eyes to check the time. When you have finished sit quietly for several minutes without opening your eyes. Then open your eyes, but remain seated for a while longer before you stand up. Do not stand up too suddenly after you have finished the practice.

Note: With all new experiences there will be a settling-in period. Do not worry if you find distracting thoughts entering your mind. Concentrate on the exhalation and the word 'one'. After a while you will be relaxing successfully. Once you have mastered the response, and this should not take long, practise it once or twice daily.

Autogenic training

This relaxation technique developed out of studies on hypnosis made at the early part of this century. The founder, Dr Johannes Heinrich Schultz, noticed that people under hypnosis experienced a peculiar heaviness in their limbs and an accompanying feeling of warmth as they relaxed. He argued that if this,

what he called 'central shift', could be brought about voluntarily by individuals, then they would be able to hypnotize themselves into a state of complete relaxation, and hence, while undergoing the experience, ease many of the tensions under which they were suffering.

In 1932 he published his thesis, *Autogenic Training, Concentrative Self-Relaxation,* which has ever since been the basis of this self-generating method of relaxation. One of Shultz's disciples, Dr Hannes Lindemann, who survived a 72-day solo crossing of the Atlantic in a canvas canoe in 1957, claimed that he was able to cope with the stresses of such a trip because he used autogenic training. Indeed, Lindemann had been taught by Schultz.

The benefits of this technique, like those of many others, not only apply to mental stress, but it is claimed that many physical disorders can be alleviated, if not cured, by this training.

Our four basic elements still apply here. It is recommended that a sitting position be used, and that whenever you apply the technique you do not allow a too strongly willed approach to interfere with the natural occurrence of relaxation. It is believed that in forcing yourself to relax you set up opposite impulses which cancel the effect you are striving for. This is not to say that you must not strongly believe that success will come. It is recommended that you do the exercises for about 10 minutes three times daily. Here is the full sequence of exercises; you should progress from one to the other according to the advice given. It is advisable to check with your own doctor about the heart exercise if you have any history of cardiac malfunction.

It is important that at the end of every exercise session, whether you have experienced any sensation of heaviness and warmth or not, you must terminate the session in a positive way. Say to yourself, 'stretch and bend arms, breathe deeply and open eyes.' As you say this, bend and stretch the arms vigorously several times.

1 Inducing heaviness

Once in a comfortable position say to yourself:
— 'My right (left) arm is heavy.'
Concentrate on your dominant arm. Repeat the formula about 6 times. If distraction hinders your efforts, start again, and concentrate on the training formula. Once you experience the heaviness, say to yourself, 'I am completely calm', then repeat the heaviness formula. All this should take about a minute. Repeat the formula about 18 times during every exercise in the first week.

2 The 'warmth' exercise

This exercise, which is aimed at relaxing the blood vessels, should be attempted after about two weeks of training, whether you have experienced heaviness or not. Most people experience heaviness very quickly. The new formula is:

— 'My right (left) arm is very warm.'

The following exercise then applies:

— 'I am completely calm.' (once)
— 'The right arm is very heavy.' (about 6 times)
— 'I am completely calm.' (once)
— 'The right arm is very warm.' (about 6 times)
— 'I am completely calm.' (once)
— 'The right arm is very warm.' (6 to 12 times)

Termination: 'Stretch and bend arms, breathe deeply, open eyes.'

The feelings of heaviness and warmth eventually spread to the whole of the body and a sensation of great relaxation is experienced.

3 The heart exercise

(Omit this if it is medically unsuitable for you.) The heaviness and warmth exercises which result in a 'relaxation' of blood vessels seems to mean that more blood and oxygen goes to the heart, thereby relieving it of some pains. This would seem to make sense; if there is less peripheral demand, then the heart must benefit.

The new formula is:

— 'My heart beats calmly and strongly.'

The following exercise then applies:

— 'I am completely calm.' (once)
— 'My right arm is very heavy.' (6 times)
— 'I am completely calm.' (once)
— 'My right arm is very warm.' (6 times)
— 'I am completely calm.' (once)
— 'My heart beats calmly and strongly.' (6 times)
— 'I am completely calm.' (once)

Termination: 'Stretch and bend arms, breathe deeply, open eyes.'

4 The breathing exercise

Many people find that after only two or three training sessions their breathing becomes calmer and more regular. Since there is a direct relationship between breathing and heart rate, if your heart is beating regularly, then you will be breathing regularly. Therefore we recommend that the breathing exercise can be done instead of the heart exercise.

The new formula is:

— 'My breathing is calm and regular.'

The following exercise then applies:

— 'I am completely calm.' (once)
— 'My right arm is very heavy.' (6 times)

— 'I am completely calm.' (once)
— 'My right arm is very warm.' (6 times)
— 'I am completely calm.' (once)
— 'My heart beats calmly and strongly.' (6 times)
— 'I am completely calm.' (once)
— 'My breathing is calm and regular.' (6 times)

Termination: 'Stretch and bend arms, breathe deeply, open eyes.'

5 The abdominal exercise

Relaxation of the abdomen, the release of tension which we know as a 'tightening of the stomach', is a major achievement for any relaxation technique. The sensitive bundle of nerves known as the solar plexus controls the responses of the stomach organs to various stimuli. Logically, then, in our attempt to relax all parts of the body the abdominal exercise comes next.

The formula is:

— 'Abdomen flowingly warm.'

The following exercise then applies:

— 'I am completely calm.' (once)
— 'My right arm is very heavy.' (6 times)
— 'I am completely calm.' (once)
— 'My right arm is very warm.' (6 times)
— 'I am completely calm.' (once)
— 'My heart beats calmly and strongly.' (6 times)
— 'I am completely calm.' (once)
— 'My breathing is calm and regular.' (6 times)
— 'I am completely calm.' (once)
— 'Abdomen flowingly warm.' (6 times)

Termination: 'Stretch and bend arms, breathe deeply, open eyes.'

6 The head exercise

This is the final exercise.

The new formula is:

— 'Forehead pleasantly cool.'

The following exercise then applies:

— 'I am completely calm.' (once)
— 'My right arm is very heavy.' (6 times)
— 'I am completely calm.' (once)
— 'My right arm is very warm.' (6 times)
— 'I am completely calm.' (once)
— 'My heart beats calmly and strongly.' (6 times)
— 'I am completely calm.' (once)
— 'My breathing is calm and regular.' (6 times)
— 'I am completely calm.' (once)
— 'Abdomen flowingly warm.' (6 times)
— 'I am completely calm.' (once)
— 'Forehead pleasantly cool.' (6 times)
— 'I am completely calm.' (once)

Termination: 'Stretch and bend arms, breathe deeply, open eyes.'.

Note: Success with this technique will come only with systematic practice. Spend about two weeks trying to get the feeling of heaviness before trying to instil the feeling of warmth. Thereafter progress at your own pace. It may take several months before you can complete the whole schedule successfully. Once you have become familiar with the formulae you will find that you can abbreviate them thus:
— 'Calm – heaviness – warmth.'
— 'Heart and breathing completely calm.'
— 'Abdomen flowingly warm.'
— 'Forehead pleasantly cool.'
Termination: 'Stretch and bend arms, breathe deeply, open eyes.'

Progressive relaxation

One cannot progress far into the field of mental relaxation techniques without invoking the name and work of Dr Edmund Jacobson. As long ago as 1909 Dr Jacobson noticed that even when a person was ostensibly at rest, there was residual tension in the muscle fibres. He invented a device, the integrating neurovoltmeter, to measure the amount of electrical activity there was in the apparently resting muscle. In 1929 this eminent physiologist and medical practitioner wrote a book called *Progressive Relaxation*, in which he set out his theories — all of which were scientifically validated — and in which he set out a series of exercises. Forty-six years later he was still publishing on the same subject, and still practising medicine. Throughout the last sixty years Dr Jacobson's techniques have been widely used to combat a whole series of physical ailments as well as a range of mental disorders.

For our basic progressive relaxation course a daily session of about three quarters of an hour is suggested. Remember, as with all relaxation techniques, undue effort or tension on your part will be self-defeating. This course aims at reducing muscular stress initially, and, hence, allowing the complex chemical behaviour of the body a 'breather' (bearing in mind the relationship between the physiology and psychology of the body).

Wear comfortably loose clothing and choose a quiet semi-darkened room in which to relax. Lie down on a bed or sofa so that no muscle groups are supporting themselves. You must be completely supported by the bed. Relax as much as you can. Your weight should sink into the bed. Now tense the muscles of your forearms very gradually. Don't move the arms. Some practitioners advocate that you also make a fist — others don't. Hold your arms stiff for about 10 seconds, then stiffen your arms a little more. Hold for another 10 seconds. Notice

how your arms are feeling. They will seem taut, perhaps a little sore. The first successful progressive relaxation is to be able to recognize what your muscles feel like when they are tense.

Now let your arms gradually relax, and notice the different sensation as they do so. Concentrate only on the arms. Try not to allow tensing to occur in other regions. Once relaxed, stay that way for 2 to 3 minutes. Repeat this process three times, holding on to the tension a little longer each time so that on the third repetition you contract the muscles for 30 seconds. The more practised you become the more you will notice that the residual tension diminishes. Now repeat the same procedure with the other muscle groups. Thus:

Forehead, upper face, jaw, neck
— Raise the eyebrows and frown. Hold for 10 seconds, relax and repeat as for the arms.
— Wrinkle the nose and shut your eyelids tightly. Hold and repeat as above.
— Clench the jaw, pull back the corners of your mouth and force the tongue into the roof of your mouth. Relax and repeat as before.
— Pull your chin down onto your chest at the same time as you pull the head back with the muscles at the back of the neck. Relax and repeat as before.

Shoulders and upper back
— Pull back your shoulder blades as if you wanted them to meet in the middle. At the same time try and touch your shoulders to your ears. Relax and repeat as before.

Stomach
— Tense your stomach muscles by pulling the stomach inwards and pressing the muscles downwards. Hold, relax, repeat as before.

Legs
— Tense your thigh muscles, relax and repeat.
— Bend your toes towards your shins so that the calf muscles are tensed. Relax and repeat as before.

Note: You should progress with all the exercises as you did with the arms and hands. After a while you should be able to dispense with the initial tensing and go straight into the deeply relaxed state. The object of the tensing is so that you can feel what tension is really like.

Some people prefer to relax completely after each bout of muscle contraction. You may like to experiment to see which method gives you a greater awareness of deep relaxation.

You may also find it of benefit to start each

session with a few deep breaths. Many people prefer Dr Jacobson's method of concentrating on a symbol or sound, what is known as a *mantra*. You must choose your own method to suit yourself.

Biofeedback

Biofeedback is the name given to the use of machines to monitor certain bodily functions. For example, the electromyograph (EMG) or the electrocardiograph (ECG) are machines which feed back biological information about, in the case of the ECG, the heart. From the information received the physician is able to make accurate diagnoses and prescribe appropriate treatment. There is a growing use of different types of machines by individuals for the purpose of controlling what have hitherto been regarded as involuntary functions. In principle the machines send back information to the individual about, for example, whether he is too tense, so that eventually the information will be monitored by the individual himself without the use of the machine. The old fashioned lie-detector is one such machine.

Before listing some of the machines on the market, we think it appropriate to say that the indiscriminate use of biofeedback machines is unwise. There is a possibility that a machine could feed back incorrect information; researchers in New York found that certain nervous twitching fed back the same information that desirable brain waves did. Thus the users of the machine, happy to think that the electrical activity in the brain was relaxed and 'normal' trained themselves to become prize twitchers! As the aim of these machines is to get you to adapt desirably your harmful behaviour you must exercise caution in the use of them.

On the positive side many large corporations are using biofeedback techniques to monitor staff voluntarily, and are finding that the resultant greater relaxation of their employees is proving economically successful. For the individuals, too, job satisfaction seems greater, the desire for promotion and responsibility but without tension is increasing, and labour relations generally are taking a turn for the better.

Galvanic skin response (GSR)

This machine measures skin resistance to mild electric currents. Electrodes are attached to the fingertips and either on a dial or by a rise in feedback tone the level of skin resistance is measured. The more tense and anxious a person is the lower will be the skin resistance. It is possible with the use of this machine to lower one's own tension and increase one's relaxation. If the machine has a buzzer attached then as one is linked with it the reduction in pitch of the buzz allows one to listen to, as well as otherwise

experience, a reduction in stress. Once one knows what relaxation feels like, one can adapt one's subsequent behaviour accordingly.

Electrothermal machine

This machine detects changes in peripheral skin temperature. The temperature of the fingertips is associated with the activity of the smooth muscles in the peripheral arteries. If one is tense, the arteries contract. If one is relaxed, they dilate. This biofeedback information is used in, among other things, the treatment of migraines.

Electroencephalograph (EEG)

The EEG machine picks up and reports back on the electrical activity in the brain's cortex. Electrodes are attached to the scalp and a paper trace charts brain wave patterns. Certain patterns are associated with certain states of mind, and without going into details we would state that the alpha rhythms are the ones sought in training.

Electromyograph (EMG)

Just as the brain generates electrical impulses, so does muscle tissue. The EMG measures muscular tension; electrodes are placed on the forearm, for example, and sound or lights are sent back to indicate the degree of tension in the individual.

Note: All these machines have the advantage that, if used properly, they are a means of drug-free self-help for any individual. They can be used in conjunction with other relaxation techniques and are already successful in treating hypertension, migraines and stomach disorders. It is possible in the future that individuals will be able to control their own blood pressure and even their own cardio-respiratory systems by detecting early warning signs of impending trouble.

Transcendental meditation (TM)

Arguably this relaxation technique is the best-known of all. We recommend the principles of TM but are in no way concerned with any other cultic or mystical association it may have. Before we suggest a simple way of putting it into practice there are certain important things which should be said.

There are no degrees in meditation. You can neither meditate 'well' nor meditate 'badly'. You are either meditating or you are not. For many Westerners the habit of meditation does not come easily; we are accustomed to continual activity, and the concept of sitting down and 'doing nothing' for a period of time is foreign to our culture. If you wish to practise meditation it is important from the outset that you realize the habit will not come easily. You must persevere with it rather than work at it.

On the positive side remind yourself of the objective you have in mind. You are seeking to relax mental and physical activity at certain times of the day at the same time as you are re-thinking your daily lifestyle. You are doing this while adjusting your dietary, smoking and exercise habits, all for the aim of reducing the risk of cardiac and associated diseases. It is a proven fact that meditation lowers the respiration rate, lowers skin resistance to electrical current, causes the brain waves to become regular and synchronized, generally slows down the metabolic rate of the body and gives a feeling of peace and warmth. And all the while the mind is still alert. These are convincing advantages, are they not?

In order to do transcendental meditation you should choose a quiet, semi-darkened environment where you can remain undisturbed for about 20 minutes. Sit in a comfortable position, preferably with your back being supported. Wear comfortable, loose-fitting clothes. Allow your breathing to relax; let it find its own rhythm. Now concentrate on your breathing and on nothing else. Be aware of your chest and stomach movements. At this point bring in the meditative object, the *mantra*. As you inhale say to yourself the word 'in'. As you exhale say to yourself the word 'out'. Say the words 'in' and 'out' on each inhalation and exhalation respectively. While you are concentrating on them no alien thoughts should enter your consciousness. If you find it difficult to concentrate remind yourself of what you are aiming at. Re-read all we have said about stress and relaxation. Concentrate again on your breathing. Meditate like this twice a day for about 20 minutes.

If you find this technique not to your liking try any of the others below. Instead of concentrating on the words 'in' and 'out', forget the breathing and change the *mantra;* use *om* or *ram*, both Sanskrit words, and meaningless to us. Say the *mantra* over and over to yourself. Vary the pitch and tone of the word. Sometimes extend its length, at others say it quickly and repeatedly.

If you prefer to meditate with your eyes open focus on an object in your meditation room such as a flower or ornament. Concentrate on the appeal the object has to your vision. Forget about the physical sensation of breathing. Remembering all the time that there will, in the early stages, be obtrusive thoughts bombarding your consciousness. Try to eliminate them by concentrating on your *mantra*. Don't let the obtrusive thoughts cause you distress. Like any other skill, meditation is specific and acquired.

A final word

Of the techniques mentioned briefly in this chapter we would recommend no one method as better than another. The aims for all are the same. The measurable beneficial results of each are encouragingly alike. In the last resort you will decide which method suits you. What we do guarantee is that training in mental relaxation techniques will increase your life expectancy, will reduce the levels of stress you experience and will give you a sense of well-being and serenity that you have probably not experienced before.

3 Diet and nutrition

Weight problems

There can be no doubt that there is a link between coronary heart disease, diet and obesity; and it is for this reason that a study of diet and general sound nutrition should be made. Because the whole field of nutrition and dietetics is one of the least understood and most abused as far as the average person is concerned, this chapter aims to explain the reasons for obesity, its effects, how it may be reduced and give the reader an understanding of good nutrition, so that he can immediately apply this knowledge to his benefit.

Let us now look in more detail at obesity as a factor in coronary heart disease and its detrimental effects on other aspects of health. Here are some facts about obesity of which you may not be aware.

1 Overweight people are twice as likely to have symptoms of chronic illness than those who are not.
2 Overweight people are often out of breath and may suffer from overtiredness, constipation, headaches and indigestion.
3 Overweight people are more prone to arthritis, diabetes, high blood pressure, hernias, varicose veins, haemarrhoids, gastric and duodenal ulcers, diverticulitis and diseases of the liver and kidneys.
4 Overweight people run four times the risk of dying during surgical operations under general anaesthetic than people of normal weight. Even after surgery, the rate of healing is slower, convalescence is delayed and the chances of complications such as pneumonia and deep venous thrombosis are greater.
5 Overweight women are more likely to be infertile than those of normal weight. When they do conceive, they are more likely to suffer complications such as varicose veins and toxaemia of pregnancy.
6 Insurance companies, who possess the most complete statistics relating to health and mortality, calculate that overweight people have five times the chance of suffering from heart disease and, as a result, the insurance premiums are usually higher.

7 Overweight people are not as tolerated by our society as they used to be. They are now figures of fun, people who have difficulty finding clothes that fit, who perspire with the slightest activity, who cannot enjoy rough and tumble games with their children without getting out of breath and who become gradually more and more self-conscious about their condition causing themselves and their families worry and distress.

These are some of the effects of obesity upon the average person. But how does one decide whether one is obese?. The usual way is by referring to a weight table, which gives the average or desirable weights (which are not the same thing) for a given height and build. Obesity has been defined as the state of an individual who weighs 10 per cent above his standard weight, but this may not be a satisfactory criterion. An athlete may well be 'overweight' but certainly not obese, while a sedentary individual with a small frame and poorly developed muscles may be obese without being overweight. But, if you remember the inaccuracies that may occur, and use the tables accordingly, it is possible to get a good idea of whether you are overweight or not. To this purpose, we have reproduced such a table of desirable weights for men and women here. Note that the weights given are for when clothed.

However, probably the best method is the least scientific. Stand naked in front of a full-length mirror and take a long critical look at yourself. Some authorities recommend jumping up and down and seeing whether anything wobbles that shouldn't! Most people will be able to tell immediately if they are overweight and, more than likely, confirm a thought that had been at the back of their minds for some time.

Some causes of overweight

Having decided that one is overweight to some extent, let us see how this state of affairs was reached. Many researchers have demonstrated a whole range of disorders of the metabolism in overweight individuals. When obesity has existed for some time, insensitivity develops to the control of the levels of fat in the blood. This interferes with the action of

27

insulin, which prevents the proper use of blood sugar by the body. This leads to a reduction in the metabolic rate, and so the fat is used up more slowly, hence a vicious circle. Excess fat makes for good insulation, so less energy needs to be expended to keep warm. Increased weight leads to lessened physical activity. The above factors, however, contribute to the maintenance of obesity rather than to its cause. The basic cause of obesity can be simply defined as due to the energy input in the form of food being greater than the energy output in the form of activity.

Certain factors may influence obesity. It can easily be seen that being overweight does tend to run

Fig. 2 Desirable weights for men and women

According to height and frame. Ages 25 and over.

Height in shoes	Weight and pounds (in indoor clothing)		
	Small frame	Medium frame	Large frame
	Men		
5ft 2 inches	112-120	118-129	126-141
3	115-123	121-133	129-144
4	118-126	124-136	132-148
5	121-129	127-139	135-152
6	124-133	130-143	138-156
7	128-137	134-147	142-161
8	132-141	138-152	147-166
9	136-145	142-156	151-170
10	140-150	146-160	155-174
11	144-154	150-165	159-179
6 ft 0 inches	148-158	154-170	164-184
1	152-162	158-175	168-189
2	156-167	162-180	173-194
3	160-171	167-185	178-199
4	164-175	172-190	182-204
	Women		
4 ft 10 inches	92-98	96-107	104-119
11	94-101	98-110	106-122
5ft 0 inches	96-104	101-113	109-125
1	99-107	104-116	112-128
2	102-110	107-119	115-131
3	105-113	110-122	118-134
4	108-116	113-126	121-138
5	111-119	116-130	125-142
6	114-123	120-135	129-146
7	118-127	124-139	133-150
8	122-131	128-143	137-154
9	126-135	132-147	141-158
10	130-140	136-151	145-163
11	134-144	140-155	149-168
6ft 0 inches	138-148	144-159	153-173

in families. Studies in the United States have shown that:
- In families with normal parents, less than 10 per cent of children are obese.
- In families with one parent obese, approximately 45 per cent of children are obese.
- In families with both parents obese, approximately 80 per cent of children are obese.

This could well be due to family eating habits, although some studies seem to indicate that a genetic factor may be present.

Physical activity today is much less than it used to be due to many factors, including mechanized transport, increased automation and shorter working hours. In contrast to the lack of activity, food intake seems to be increasing. This too has many causes, including more intensive farming methods, more money to spend, more leisure time and anxiety eating. The overweight are not necessarily big meal eaters, often they are between-meal nibblers or night eaters. Weight can increase without gross over-eating. A sedentary individual weighting 11 stones 10 pounds can put on 13 pounds in five years by eating only ¾ ounces of sugar daily, or half that amount of butter, above the body's needs.

A great many people manage to maintain a reasonably stable weight throughout their entire lives without needing to think about their diet. This suggests some efficient, built-in system of controlling food intake. Many theories have been advanced to explain this phenomenon, but none is entirely satisfactory. One of these theories is based on the fact that some individuals consume much more energy than others in the performance of the same task. Hormonal and metabolic differences could be responsible.

An interesting approach to the problem of obesity was made by Cleave and Campbell in their book *Diabetes, Coronary Thrombosis and the Saccharine Disease*. The -rine ending is pronounced like the river Rhine and 'saccharine' thus means related to sugar, and is not anything to do with the artificial sweetener. In this book, these eminently qualified doctors reasoned that the cause of obesity was due to the refining process to which most starches are subject. This process causes a removal of the filling roughage from the food, while at the same time, the relative proportion of starch is increased. This unnatural concentration of starch tends to deceive the tongue and appetite, and over-eating occurs. This theory rather neatly explains why obesity is so rare in primitive societies and non-existent in wild animals. We certainly cannot blame merely an excess of food, because Nature's answer to that is

an increase in population and not overweight. The refining of carbohydrates is also responsible for other problems, such as chronic constipation, diverticular disease and, some experts believe, cancer of the bowel. Refined food also contains less nutrients; for example, white flour contains very little of the chromium, zinc, iron, manganese, B vitamins and vitamin E present in the whole grain. A famous nutritionist once said that there were more nutrients in the packaging of a box of cornflakes than in its contents!

Before we consider what can be done to reduce weight, it would be useful for us to consider some of the principles upon which nutrition is based, so that we can better understand the application of those principles in the latter part of this chapter.

Energy

The word 'calorie' is one which we hear time and time again, particularly in relation to slimming. But to many people the calorie is an incantation invoked by a wife or lady friend when looking at a menu in a restaurant; for example, 'I shouldn't really have the Black Forest gateau, it has so many calories!' This tends to leave us with the impression that the more calories a food has, the more desirable it suddenly becomes. Which, in an illogical way, is not so far removed from the truth.

In fact, the calorie is no more than a unit in which energy can be measured. When Sir Isaac Newton formulated his famous Laws of Thermodynamics, he made a number of fundamental statements concerning energy. For our purposes, it is only necessary to know that Newton showed that energy cannot be created nor destoryed, but it can be changed from one form into another.

The prime source of energy on this planet is the breakdown of matter in the Sun. This travels to Earth in the form of solar energy. Plants are able to trap this energy directly by converting it into chemical energy in the form of starch, a stable chemical substance. This store of energy can then be utilized by the animal kingdom, and the consumption of plants is the source of energy for the majority of animals. But even in plants uneaten by animals this stored energy does not disappear. For example, coal and oil are the results of the transformation of the energy of prehistoric plants.

Every action performed by the living body requires energy, and the production of each drop of saliva, digestive juice, urine or sweat requires energy, besides the more obvious actions such as movement and growth. Thus Man's energy is obtained from the Sun indirectly via the vegetable kingdom, either by eating plants, or by eating animals that eat plants.

Although energy is interconvertible, the conversion from one form to another, particularly chemical into mechanical, is never an efficient process, with most of the energy being lost as heat. The car engine is a good example of this, with chemical energy in the form of petrol or diesel oil being turned into mechanical energy or motion, and with a large amount of waste heat being produced. There is certainly enough heat produced to melt metal, as anyone whose engine has siezed up through lack of oil can testify. In fact, the comparison between Man and the engine is quite apt, in that both are approximately 25 per cent efficient. In Man, this heat is used to maintain the temperature of the body, but unless the external environment is extremely cold, only a small amount of the heat produced is needed for this purpose, and the remainder is given off into the atmosphere. Calculations show that ten people sitting quietly and comfortably give off the same amount of heat as a one-bar electric fire. The more active they become, the greater the amount of heat they produce.

In practice, it is convenient to measure the energy output of the body in terms of the heat produced, because as we have just seen, the two are directly related.

The calorie unmasked!

The units for measuring this heat are calories. In nutrition, the amounts measured are relatively large and so we use the kilocalorie, or Calorie with a capital C, which is 1000 times bigger than the physicist's calorie. However, common usage has resulted in the Calorie being spelt with a small c and we will continue to use this form in order to avoid confusion.

In order to find out more about the heat loss from the body, a room was built in which a person lived for a number of days performing various activities, and the heat produced was measured. It was through these experiments that the rate of energy expenditure while performing different tasks was first accurately measured.

If we examine in detail the amount of calories expended performing various tasks, we can then calculate with a reasonable degree of accuracy the total amount of calories used during a 24-hour period. Let us examine the amount of energy used by a sedentary worker; for example, a clerk or, for that matter, a senior executive.

	Total calories
8 hours in bed	500
8 hours at work, comprising of	
5 hrs mostly sitting (1.5 cal./min.)	450
3 hrs standing, walking etc. (2.5 cal./min.)	450

8 hours non-occupational activities, i.e.	
1 hr washing, dressing (3.5 cal./min.)	210
1 hr walking (4.2 cal./min.)	250
4 hrs sitting (1.4 cal./min.)	340
1½ hrs gardening (5.0 cal./min.)	450
1½ hrs domestic chores (1.7 cal./min.)	50
Total	2700

Thus we can see that the energy expenditure of our imaginary individual is 2700 calories per day.

If the same calculations are performed for moderately active people, such as workers in light industry, postmen, bus conductors, etc., we find that their energy expenditure is about 3000 calories daily. Very active people such as foundry workers, coal face workers and army recruits can expend a total of 3600 calories each day. It may come as a surprise that sedentary workers include such diverse people as office workers, pilots, teachers, journalists, architects, clergy, doctors, lawyers and shop workers. There are no class barriers when it comes to spending energy!

We described earlier how energy cannot be created or destroyed, therefore the energy that comes out of the body had to come in from somewhere, and the only way it can come in is in the way of food. It is possible to obtain accurate values of the calories found in different foods. With this information we can compare the energy imput in the form of food, against the energy output in the form of work done. If an individual consumes food to the value of 3000 calories and uses up 2600 calories during that day, 400 calories are left over. It is these calories which are stored as fat and over a long period of time cause obesity. If a smaller amount of calories is consumed than is used, the body burns the necessary amount of fat to balance the equation and the individual loses weight.

Nutrition

Now that we have established some of the causes of overweight and looked at the way in which a quantitative check can be kept on energy output in the form of calories, we turn our attention to the energy input, i.e. food. This will involve us in a brief look at the history of nutrition and the structure of a sound diet. We can then look at how this diet can be modified to ensure that obesity is controlled and health restored.

Nutrition can be defined as the relationship between the food eaten and the person eating it. Proper nutrition implies that adequate amounts of food of sufficient quality are being received by the body so that it is obtaining all the essential nutrients, i.e. carbohydrates for energy, proteins for growth and repair, fats for structure and energy, and minerals and vitamins, which act together with the other nutrients to maintain the health and integrity of the body. A lack of any one or more of these components in the diet, or a loss of their quality, or an inability by the body to absorb them from the intestine, may produce no immediate signs of ill-health. However, if the process continues, a gradual decline in the health of the individual will become apparent, and in many cases may eventually lead to serious disease or even death. At the same time, the opposite is also true. It is possible to cause serious harm to the body by taking in excessive amounts of most of the individual nutrients. For example, a long-term, above-average intake of iron can lead to irreversible liver damage, while large doses of Vitamins A and D have also been shown to be responsible for disturbances in body function.

Man's knowledge of nutrition as a science is relatively recent. That is not to say, however, that the relationship between food and disease is also recent knowledge. Hippocrates, the father of medicine, was the author of a book which discussed the merits of certain foods and their effects on the healthy and diseased individual. However, many of his principles wcrc based upon the philosophies popular at that time, and upon a total misunderstanding of the anatomy and physiology of the body. But we should remember that this book was written more than 400 years BC!

Looking at the works of the Roman and early English authors we see no advances, and, on the whole, this state of affairs continued right up to the mid-eighteenth century, when the science of chemistry began to make strides forward. It was at about this time that the effects of deficient diets for long periods of time were beginning to cause concern, particularly in the Royal Navy, where at any one time, at least 50 per cent of a ship's crew were unfit for duty because of scurvy, a deficiency disease caused by a lack of Vitamin C. The addition of fresh fruit and vegetables to the sailors' diet eliminated scurvy and this has often been given as the reason for Britain's supremacy at sea. However, this feat of nutrition was not performed by scientists, but by the great sailors, explorers and observers such as Captain Cook.

Up to relatively recent times, research had been primarily directed at the effects of a lack of food or a factor in that food on the body and it was through such research and experiments on humans and animals that the vitamins were isolated. At the same time, the importance of minerals such as calcium and iron was gradually becoming apparent. As a result, it is now possible to draw up lists of all the known nutrients, giving their functions and the requirements of them by the body for health. This list is by no means complete, and numerous substances are waiting to be evaluated.

It is only in the last twenty-five years or less, however, that we have started to take an active interest in the effects of overnutrition. Certainly, most people knew that if you ate too much you became fat, but beyond that lay a grey area about which little was known. As time went on, arguments raged between different factions of scientists: some claimed that the sole cause of heart disease was a high calorie intake, others blamed diets high in animal fats and cholesterol, while still others looked for one vitamin or trace element, the absence of which caused heart disease. Certainly the absence of some nutrients or the excess of others can be demonstrated in many patients with heart disease, but it does seem rather too simple to expect that one factor only could be the cause of a condition which claimed more lives in the United States than any other.

Independent researchers have, more recently, been looking at the effects of technology upon the quality of food. Modern foods usually contain at least one or two, if not more, of the following additives: preservatives, antioxidants, antibiotics, hormones, stabilizers, emulsifiers, coloring and flavouring chemicals, bleaches, extenders, thickeners, curing agents and sweeteners. Most, if not all, have no nutritive value; in fact, more are used to disguise cheap, poor quality ingredients, or to make them more palatable than they really are. Many of the additives first used have now been withdrawn because they have been shown to be harmful, causing anything from skin rashes to cancer. As time passes, many of those additives generally regarded as safe today are bound to be proved hazardous. Even now, some doctors are proving that people can be allergic to many of these additives, and suffering from often incapacitating illnesses because of them. Needless to say, this claim has been rejected out of hand by the food industry.

Let us now look at the components of the normal diet individually, beginning with the carbohydrates.

Carbohydrates

These are the chief source of the energy upon which all the functions of the body are based. They are a group of apparently unrelated substances, such as sugars, starches and cellulose. However, the basic unit that makes up all these substances is a fairly simple structure containing only carbon, hydrogen and oxygen. This unit is called a simple sugar or monosaccharide, of which the most important is glucose. Table sugar, or sucrose, is made up of two such simple sugars, glucose and fructose linked together, while starch is made up of very long chains of glucose molecules. In addition to the sugars and starches, which are available to the body, there are also other forms which the body cannot utilize. These are the celluloses which make up the 'skeleton' of the plant, and they are indigestible to Man. They do, however, serve an essential purpose in the diet as they form the roughage or fibre in the diet that helps move the meal through the digestive system. A lack of this fibre has only recently been officially acclaimed by the medical profession as a major factor in constipation, and, as we have seen earlier, others take the effects of a lack of fibre still further, and link it with the onset of diseases such as obesity, diabetes, diverticular disease and cancer of the bowel.

In the process of digestion, all of the available carbohydrate is reduced into its constituent units of simple sugars, by far the most important of which is glucose. This is absorbed through the intestine into the bloodstream, from which it is taken up by the cells of the body and quickly used as fuel by tissues such as the brain, nervous systems and the muscles. A small proportion of the remaining glucose is converted into glycogen, another carbohydrate, and stored in the liver and muscles. This can be looked upon as a short-term store, rather like a float in a cash register, which under normal circumstances should remain relatively constant, although the units which make it up may be changing, but under unusual conditions, it may be spent without immediately causing distress. The rest of the absorbed glucose is converted into fat and stored in special cells, where it acts as a long-term store; or, to continue our financial analogy, a bank account, in which the energy can be kept out of the way, but is available within a relatively short space of time to spend when times are hard.

From the point of view of dietary sources, we can be sure that on any average diet, our intake of carbohydrates will be sufficient. They are found in the form of sugars in fruits, and as starch in root vegetables such as potatoes, in seeds, grains and bulbs, such as onions and leeks.

The carbohydrates, as a group, have probably come in for more criticism and controversy than any other food. We have already studied Cleave and Campbell's objection to the refined carbohydrates which is based on the fact that the refining process concentrates the carbohydrate so that we can consume amounts out of all proportions to what we could eat in the natural form. For example, to eat the equivalent of one gram of sugar, we would have to consume seven times that weight of apples, fourteen times that of broccoli, and five times that of cooked peas or potato. At the same time, while sugar contains no other nutrients, all the other foods contain protein, vitamins and minerals. In this way, sugar can replace more nutritious foods in the diet, while at the same time, causing deficiencies to develop and placing a strain on the digestive system. Sugar can also create a form of addiction because of the speed at which it enters the blood. This creates a short-lived feeling of well-being followed by a sensation of fatigue which creates a desire for something sweet. It is this reaction that causes more diets to be broken than anything else. Those of us not endowed with a cast-iron will and self control, and who have tried to diet before, will know just how strong those cravings can be. One way to avoid this reaction is to eat smaller meals at more frequent intervals.

Proteins
The second food class is comprised of the proteins. These are some of the more important elements in the maintenance of good health. Proteins are essential for the formation of the structure of the body, and also form a part of the molecules of hormones and enzymes. But unlike carbohydrates and fats, the body appears to have no significant store of protein, so a regular dietary intake is essential.

Proteins are broken down by digestion into their simplest components, called amino acids. There are approximately twenty of these amino acids found in the proteins in the diet, and the body needs a constant supply to replace those that it loses. Not every food contains all of these amino acids, but the body is able to form all the amino acids given a supply of only eight specific ones which are called the essential amino acids. However, without even one of the eight, protein synthesis will slow or even stop. Thus a protein food is only as good as its lowest, or limiting, amino acid.

Protein-containing foods are often categorized into first- or second-class proteins depending on whether or not they contain all eight essential amino acids in the right proportions. Most meats and dairy produce are complete proteins, as are eggs, while most beans and cereals, which can contain high proportions of protein, tend to be incomplete. However, a vegetarian can balance his diet quite easily by combining these second-class proteins in the right way, particularly if he takes a little dairy produce and uses common sense.

When supplies of carbohydrates in the body are low, proteins can be broken down in the body into energy. However, they cannot be broken down completely and the remaining waste products are then excreted from the bloodstream by the kidneys into the urine. If the kidneys are damaged or overworked, or if there is a lot of waste to be got rid of, some of it may accumulate in the tissues and joints forming crystals, and producing in some individuals the condition known as gout. This can occur in people who try a high protein, low carbohydrate diet for too long, or without any supervision.

So, although a diet containing adequate protein is essential, and the quality of the protein has to be high, excessive intake may be harmful. From the point of view of health, in fact, a vegetarian diet, or a day or two weekly without meat, has a lot to offer. Medical research in the United States has shown strong evidence that the incidence of heart disease, high blood pressure, cancer of the bowel and osteoporosis (the softening of bones associated with advancing years), was much smaller in vegetarians. Needless to say, however, many societies consume a large amount of animal proteins yet enjoy a high level of health. This apparent contradiction has not yet been resolved, but it is true that most of these societies are so-called primitive, and therefore subsist mainly on whole, unrefined foods and probably get a great deal more exercise and less stress than their 'civilized' brothers!

Fats

Fats are the most concentrated form of energy in the diet and, when they are converted to energy, produce more than twice the amount of calories than can be obtained from equal weights of carbohydrate or protein. Fats have a number of important functions in the body. Some fats form, in combination with protein, the membrane which encloses each individual cell in the body. Others form a part of such essential substances as hormones and bile. Solid deposits of fat surround and protect vital organs, such as the kidneys and heart, and the layer of fat under the skin acts as an insulator against cold. Fats in the diet also act as carriers for the fat-soluble vitamins, which will be described later. So, we can see that fats are necessary for good health.

Fats can generally be divided into two types, saturated and unsaturated, depending upon the chemical structure of the fatty acids that make up the fat. Simply speaking, saturated fats are generally hard at room temperature and are derived from animal sources, e.g. lard. Unsaturated fats, including polyunsaturates, are derived from most fish oils and from vegetable, seed and nut (except coconut) sources. They are normally liquid at room temperature. The main controversy concerning fats is the relationship between saturated fats, cholesterol and heart disease.

Cholesterol is a substance related chemically to fats which is essential to the body as it forms part of the molecule of some hormones. It also forms part of the insulating membrane surrounding the nerves. When levels of cholesterol in the bloodstream are higher than average for a long time, small particles of fat and cholesterol lodge against the walls of the arteries. As more cholesterol enters the bloodstream, so these deposits become thicker, until they begin to obstruct the flow of blood. The artery becomes hard and brittle, and there is a possibility that a part of this deposit may break away into the bloodstream and lodge in an artery of the heart or brain, with fatal consequences. This hardening, known as atherosclerosis, is, as we can see elsewhere in this book, more likely to occur where there is smoking, a lack of exercise or obesity.

It was therefore thought that by removing cholesterol from the diet, the incidence of atherosclerosis would drop. A diet high in animal fats, which contain cholesterol, was suddenly frowned upon, and a sales' boom in unsaturated fats and their products occurred. However, continuing research is showing that the ability of a diet high in polyunsaturated fats to lower the blood cholesterol level is often only temporary, or, in fact, it may have no effect at all. What is more, research in a parallel direction in the United States shows that there is an apparent increase in the rate of skin cancer in people taking large quantities of vegetable fats and unsaturated oils. It is very important to stress, however, that this applies to oils extracted from their sources, and not to the consumption of foods containing polyunsaturated fats. It would seem that once the oil is extracted from its source, it becomes vulnerable to a number of damaging influences, the most important of which are heat and exposure to air, both of which seem to cancel out any benefit that a fresh oil may have had, and at the same time, create new problems.

Found in combination with cholesterol in some foods is a fat-like substance called lecithin. This appears to be able to help cholesterol and other fats to cross from the arteries into the cells where they can be utilized, thus preventing a build-up of cholesterol in the bloodstream. Eggs contain cholesterol and patients with atherosclerosis were strongly warned against eating them. However, eggs are also a good natural source of lecithin, and it can be shown that people who consume even large numbers of eggs do not usually have high blood cholesterol levels.

Even given the above information, it is still not possible to say without doubt what the relationship between fats and heart disease really is. Very often, research confirming one factor in the relationship can be contradicted by research elsewhere. We can only use the information as a guide to dietary reform.

Vitamins

The vitamins are a group of chemically unrelated substances, found in most foods, which are essential for health and well-being. They can be divided into two groups, the fat soluble, including Vitamins A, D, E and K; and the water soluble, consisting of the Vitamin B complex and Vitamin C.

Vitamin A helps to maintain the skin and the linings of the digestive tract, kidneys, bladder and lungs in good condition. It also helps to give good eyesight, particularly in dim light. Some researchers claim that Vitamin A can be effective in the reduction of high blood cholesterol levels and help to dissolve existing atherosclerosis. Vitamin A is found, preformed, in fish liver oils, liver and cheese. Vegetables, such as carrots, spinach and broccoli contain large amounts of carotene, a substance that is converted to Vitamin A in the body, hence the belief that eating carrots helped British Spitfire pilots see in the dark!

Vitamin D is a vitamin which can either be taken in food, or formed in the skin by the action of sunlight. Its most important feature is its control over the efficient laying down of calcium and phosphorus to form strong bones and teeth. There may be a relation between Vitamin D and atherosclerosis, because the body uses a derivative of cholesterol to form the vitamin in the skin, but there is no firm evidence one way or the other. Good dietary sources include fish liver oils, butter and eggs.

Vitamin E is an antioxidant; in other words, it prevents or slows the combination of oxygen with essential nutrients which make them of no use to the body. With relation to heart disease, Vitamin E is of importance in that it helps prevent the unsaturated fats and Vitamin A from breaking down or forming harmful substances when exposed to air or heat. Although there is evidence to show that a deficiency of Vitamin E can lead to increased blood cholesterol levels and atherosclerosis, recent investigations have shown that large doses tend to raise the blood pressure, especially when first taking it. The ability of Vitamin E to prevent excessive blood clotting and to reduce scar formation could be of great value in the period of recovery following a heart attack, especially if used under supervision. It is found naturally in combination with the polyunsaturated fats, in the oily portions of whole grains, seeds and beans.

Vitamin K is essential for the normal clotting mechanism of the blood. Some anticoagulant drugs (used for 'thinning' the blood) work by neutralizing this vitamin. It is normally synthesized in sufficient quantities by bacteria naturally occurring in the gut, but a course of antibiotics could kill these bacteria and cause a deficiency. Fortunately, it is also found in foods such as green plants, yoghurt, egg yolk, polyunsaturated oils and molasses.

The water soluble vitamins are more likely to be lacking in the modern diet. It is these that are dissolved out of the food by prolonged cooking, and many of them are easily broken down by heat. The Vitamin B complex comprises of seven definite members, although some authorities may include five or six other substances under the same broad heading. As a group, the members of the B complex are essential for the efficient metabolism of carbohydrates, proteins and fats. They are also needed for the correct functioning of the skin, nervous system, gastrointestinal tract, skin and liver. Two members of this complex have a direct relationship with heart disease, and appear linked to cholesterol metabolism and thus atherosclerosis. Two other substances, whose necessity is disputed by some authorities, and are included in the B complex by others, are constituents of lecithin which, as we mentioned earlier, may be a preventative factor in the build-up of blood cholesterol levels. All the B vitamins are natural constituents of brewer's yeast and liver, and most are found in whole grain cereals. The majority can be synthesized by the natural bacteria found in the healthy intestine.

Vitamin C is essential for the health and structure of the skin and blood vessels. It also acts as a natural antibiotic, thus fighting bacterial infections. It appears to be used up in vast quantities under conditions of physical or mental stress. This could be one of the ways in which stress can make a person more susceptible to illness or infection. A relationship between Vitamin C and blood cholesterol levels has been postulated, but is not widely accepted. Foods which contain Vitamin C are the citrus fruits, and most other fresh raw fruit and vegetables. This vitamin is probably the most sensitive to temperature and sunlight, so that the apparently healthy and nutritious salad and fresh fruit salad seen in a restaurant, and prepared hours earlier, may be completely deficient in Vitamin C.

Minerals

The minerals comprise the last class of nutrient essential for health. An analysis of the body shows it to comprise of relatively large amounts of calcium, chlorine, magnesium, phosphorus, potassium, sodium and sulphur. Traces of chromium, cobalt, copper, iron, fluorine, iodine, manganese, molybdenum, selenium, vanadium and zinc are also present and have demonstrable actions and effects. At the same time, small amounts of aluminium, beryllium, boron, lead, lithium, mercury, silicon, strontium and tin can be recognized by analysis; in some cases these are the results of pollution of the air, water and food, while some may have functions that science has not yet understood.

As a group, the minerals act by facilitating many biological actions in the body, including the transmission of nerve impulses, formation of red and white blood cells, and the production of hormones and enzymes. They also help to maintain the delicate balance of fluids inside and outside the cells. All of these essential minerals have to be supplied by the diet. We shall look at these very briefly, with particular reference to those minerals which are necessary for effective heart function and structure.

Calcium is primarily necessary for strong bones and teeth, but it also helps to regulate blood clotting, nerve transmission and muscle activity and appears to have a regulatory effect on the heartbeat. It is found mainly in dairy products, although cereals and grains can also act as sources.

Chromium is involved indirectly in the metabolism of glucose, fatty acids and cholesterol, as well as assisting insulin in lowering the blood sugar level. It is found in wholegrain cereals, meat and good quality brewer's yeast.

Copper is found in wholegrain cereals, liver, green leafy vegetables and dried legumes. It helps in the formation of healthy blood and bones, as well as being involved in protein metabolism.

Fluorine is found naturally in seafoods and many plants. It appears to work with calcium in the formation of healthy bones and teeth. The addition of fluorine to water, so that children's teeth are protected to some extent from decay, is an arguable practice, and enough literature, for and against, is already available, so we do not intend to discuss this further.

Iodine is essential to the body because it makes up the major part of the hormone thyroxine, which exerts its influence over every tissue of the body, by speeding up the process of metabolism. It is found in seafoods and vegetables grown in an iodine-rich soil.

Iron, found in liver, heart, lean meats and leafy green vegetables, forms the red blood pigment, haemoglobin, which carries the oxygen around the body to where it is needed. A lack of iron leads to a feeling of tiredness, and one form of anaemia.

Magnesium is found in all green leafy vegetables, wholegrain cereals and in oil-rich seeds and nuts, especially almonds. A deficiency of magnesium is thought to be closely related to coronary heart disease, because without it, blood clots may form in the heart and brain, and calcium may be deposited in the kidneys, heart and arteries, causing arteriosclerosis.

Manganese is found in wholegrain cereals, egg yolks and green vegetables. It aids in the proper utilization of cholesterol and fatty acids, as well as being responsible for activating several enzyme systems. Its lack in the diet may increase cholesterol levels in the blood.

Phosphorus is an element widely distributed in nature, and it is present in every living cell. It is found in combination with calcium as the major component of bone. Good dietary sources are meat, fish and wholegrain cereals.

Potassium is another element that is so widely distributed in Nature that, under normal circumstances, a deficiency is rare. It has many functions, most of which are affected by the balance between potassium and sodium. The normalization of the heart beat and regulation of the blood pressure are two such functions.

Sodium is also found in all living cells and the normal diet will contain enough. However, most people add excess salt to the diet and this creates an imbalance in the ratio of sodium to potassium. This is then responsible for such diverse problems as water retention, increased blood pressure, dizziness and impaired absorption of other nutrients from the intestine.

Sulphur is found in the skin, hair and nails and is responsible for their well-being. It also forms part of the insulin molecule and it plays a part in the body's utilization of energy. It is found in protein-containing foods such as meat, fish, legumes and nuts.

Vanadium is a trace element which appears to have a direct influence on cholesterol levels in the blood. It is found in seafood and in varying quantities in vegetables, depending on soil content, so seafood is probably the best source. Vanadium has been used as a supplement in order to lower blood cholesterol levels, but in large quantities it can be toxic. Diet is probably the best means of obtaining sufficient, particularly if it is sensibly balanced.

Zinc has many functions, including growth and sexual development, the proper breakdown of carbohydrate and it is also the constituent of at least twenty-five enzymes. The best sources of zinc are wholegrain cereals, some meats and seeds, and brewer's yeast.

The best sources of all mineral elements are un-refined cereals, preferably those grown on organically composted soils, organ meats, such as liver and heart, seeds, nuts and dark, leafy vegetables. The refining of cereals is largely responsible for borderline deficiencies of some trace minerals, which in turn, may be related to specific diseases.

Losing weight

By now, we should have a good knowledge of the causes and effects of obesity, and of what makes up a good balanced diet. We can now put all this information together and see how it is possible to control and banish obesity, and, at the same time, maintain a diet which will be balanced as well as healthy, thus ensuring us the maximum protection against heart disease. We have already seen that there are only two ways of losing weight: either eating less or doing more. Ways of doing more, not only for losing weight but also for improving over-all health, are fully described in the following chapters, so we will restrict ourselves here to eating less.

There are almost as many dietary regimes as there are overweight people; each one has its prophets and disciples, and each claims that it is the only way to attain smallness! In our experience, some work, but most don't. The perfect slimming diet must be inexpensive to follow, should not comprise of difficult-to-understand directions or complex calculations, it should not exclude any of the food classes, it must not depend on any commercial supplement, drug or diet aid, and it should be effortless and attractive to the person following it. If anyone knew of such a diet, he would have become rich overnight. The whole point of any diet must be to deprive the body of food to some extent, and that can never be easy. We fall into bad habits like over-eating very easily, and these habits require effort to break. Until we have made the conscious and unconscious decision to lose weight, and we realize that some inconvenience is inevitable, any diet that we embark upon is doomed to fail right from the start. The incentive that provokes determined dieting may appear insignificant: an overheard remark, a holiday snapshot showing obvious overweight, or it may be something more serious, like a failed insurance medical or symptoms of heart disease. Because of the many methods available to the prospective slimmer, we will briefly look at the main contenders.

Calorie-counting is based upon the principle that if you purposefully add up all the calories contained in your planned food intake in such a way that the intake is always made up of less calories than you expend in the day, then you must lose weight. It is possible to buy booklets containing the calorific value of virtually any food imaginable, and, for a housewife, for example, with easy access to scales and a calculator, this appears to be an easy and effective method. Even the manufacturers of convenience foods are producing low calorie meals with the calorific value printed on the package. It is not surprising to see that the manufacturers of these products also make some of the most calorie-rich foods available. The disadvantage of this method is that unless a knowledge of the principles of nutrition is held by the slimmer, a diet can be consumed which although containing the required calories, is deficient in most of the nutrients. It is also difficult to calculate accurately the number of calories in meals taken in restaurants, cafés or staff canteens.

The 'carbohydrate-unit' diet is, in some ways, easier to follow, as it lists the values of foods purely by their carbohydrate content. Its aim is to restrict the intake of carbohydrate, whilst allowing the slimmer as much meat (fatty as well as lean), cheese, butter, eggs, fats and oil as he desires. This diet, originally formulated by Professor Judkin, and the later 'Eat Fat, Grow Slim' diet of Dr Mackarness, are both based upon the premise that it is carbohydrate that is fattening, and that by restricting it, weight loss is inevitable.

The high protein, low carbohydrate diet is a regime which orignated in the United States, and is used extensively by 'Weight Watchers'. This is based upon the principle that in order for protein to be metabolized, carbohydrate must also be present. If it is not found in the diet, then the body has to convert fat stores into carbohydrate, and thus weight loss occurs. However, as we have already described, a diet high in protein, particularly animal protein, may render a person more susceptible to heart disease. This diet is also unsuitable for people with weak or damaged kidneys or liver because of the increased waste material produced during protein metabolism. It is also true that a proportion of weight loss is due to an increased loss of water, needed by the kidneys to flush out this high concentration of waste produced on this diet. As soon as the slimmer returns to a normal balanced diet, the body will retain more water, and a few pounds of extra weight reappear.

So, we can see that none of these diets is perfect. But, what is the alternative available to us? We know that in order to lose weight, we have to eat less. When we eat less, we feel hungry because a small meal will not produce the accustomed distension of the stomach, while a diet low in sugar will not give us that 'lift' that we had come to expect from our meals. To satisfy that 'still empty' feeling, a number of methods can be used. A meal high in protein or fat will remain in the stomach for longer than a sweet one, thus making us feel fuller longer, while a meal containing plenty of lightly cooked or raw vegetables and fruit, with unrefined grains, will give us a greater bulk for less calories. But all these methods are trying to maintain a condition which should not exist. They are merely treating the symptoms of obesity and over-distension, whereas they should be getting us out of the habit of over-eating, so that our over-strained stomachs can gradually regain their normal size, allowing us to feel full when we have eaten less. In the intervening time, a certain amount of hunger must be unavoidable.

The method

The following dietary outline should help all but the least determined slimmer lose weight gradually but consistently, while at the same time, maintaining a balanced intake. It must of course be remembered that every person is an individual, and will therefore respond differently to changes in his diet.

Breakfast should be a light meal. Try having fruit, such as apples, citrus fruit, pears or any other fruit in season. With this, you can have some plain yoghurt, with a little honey if absolutely necessary, although *all* sweeteners should be avoided. If you still feel hungry, try a slice of wholemeal bread, toasted if desired, with a little butter or vegetable margarine. It is surprising how filling wholemeal bread can be when compared to that white fluffy stuff some call bread. A good quality wholegrain cereal, such as Weetabix, Sunnybisk or muesli is also very satisfying and, with a few soaked dried fruits, such as apricots, prunes or sultanas, makes a nutritious, filling breakfast. Those who prefer a cooked breakfast should avoid fried food. Well-grilled bacon, poached or boiled egg with grilled tomatoes or mushrooms will make a filling meal. A disadvantage of such a meal is that it may tend to leave you lacking in mental and physical agility for a few hours until it is digested!

Try to avoid eating between meals. Snacks are never a good idea, as you never get used to having an empty stomach, and most tend to be high in sugar or carbohydrate and fat. If you are really desperate, it would be better to have something that would fill you yet not be fattening; try a piece of fruit, like an orange, or, if you are at home, a raw carrot or a stick of celery.

If you have to rely on other people's cooking for your lunch, then be careful what you choose. If lunch is your main meal, and you want a starter, choose melon, grapefruit cocktail or a clear soup, rather than pâté, pasta or fried fish. For the main course, look for grilled, steamed or boiled meat or fish rather than fried. Avoid foods in rich sauces. Have a little more of the vegetables to compensate, excluding, of course, the knob of butter and the fried potatoes or courgettes, etc. A side salad with a steak is a good choice. For dessert, something light is again best. The cheeseboard should not be considered; instead, try some water-ice, fresh fruit salad or fresh fruit.

For a lighter meal, a little lean ham, or some cheese, with a generous portion of mixed salad, is excellent. If you are making your own salad, use as many different varieties of in-season vegetables as you can. Don't be afraid to be adventurous or to use a good recipe book. Do not, however, be over-generous with the salad dressing, particularly an oily vinaigrette or salad cream. A lemon juice and herb dressing with a little olive oil can make a pleasant change. There is no reason why you can't take a prepared salad in to work with you, if you so desire.

For the evening meal, the same rules apply. If this is to be your main meal, do not eat it too late.

General points

Experiment with the whole range of vegetables and fruit. One of the main failings with a lot of diets is that they are not interesting for long enough. Remember, variety is the spice of life!

You will probably find whole foods more satisfying and tasty. A baked jacket potato looks much more than the same potato mashed. Try wholewheat pastas (available at most supermarkets), these are much more filling and appetizing than their refined counterparts, and, if used sensibly, can be included in the diet. If your previous diet contained much refined foods, you will also have the bonus of a greater feeling of well-being, more energy and all the other advantages of positive good health.

At the same time, it is sensible to steer clear of 'slimmers' foods' and other processed foods. Become a label reader and see just what your favourite snack or dish contains apart from basic ingredients; prepare to be surprised if not shocked at what you were really eating! Remember that it is usual for all ingredients to be listed in order of quantity. Note how often sugar appears high on the list, even in foods that you would never associate with sweetness. Very often, the cutting-out of all additives from a diet may lead to mild or even severe withdrawal symptoms, ranging from restlessness to headaches, nausea and other physical disturbances. This is not because your new diet is not good for you, rather your old diet was bad for you. These symptoms will pass quite soon and you will feel a sense of well-being and relaxation working its way throughout the entire body and mind.

Vegetables and clear broths can be very satisfying and nutritious, yet not at all fattening.

If you have a passion for a particular food which should not really be on the diet, it may be an idea to treat yourself to a little now and then, rather than yearning for it and eventually breaking the diet through cravings.

Avoid preparing more than you ought to eat, and then leaving the unfinished food on the table — too much temptation!

Bearing in mind all that we have learned about food, there is no reason why you can't try a low-fat or calorie-controlled diet, if you find them easier to follow. Very often, a week on a high-protein diet will give a rapid weight loss which can then be followed up by more sensible prolonged dieting.

Remember that weight loss as first can often be rapid, and then taper off depressingly. Look at long-term loss rather than daily changes. Don't weigh yourself every day; once a week is perfectly sufficient. Weigh yourself at the same time of the day each week, with empty bladder and bowel. Once at your ideal weight, try not to slide into the old bad habits. What we want you to do is not so much to follow a rigid diet, but to reform your ideas about food, so that after a time, your normal diet will consist of a balanced intake of fresh, whole, unadulterated food, your weight will remain stable and your health and appearance will continue to improve to such an extent that you will wonder how you ever managed before.

If during your diet you experience any unusual sensations, do not be unduly alarmed. During a diet, the physiology of the body alters in subtle ways, and it may be these changes that you are noticing. If they persist, or you are worried by them, seek advice.

Finally, remember that it is you who gets yourself slim. No diet will help someone who doesn't want to lose weight. Tackle the job well, and the results will be immediately obvious; make a bad job of it, and you do yourself no good, or even harm. So good luck!

4 The case against smoking

Smoking and coronary heart disease

This is the shortest chapter in the book. In terms of improving your over-all health and reducing the risk of coronary and associated disease the advice is simple. Don't smoke!

It would be inconclusive to enter the controversy about whether smoking increases the incidence of cancer; there is still too much disagreement about this among the specialists. However, it can categorically be stated that smoking does increase the risk of coronary heart disease, and certainly is the cause of much respiratory disease.

The nicotine inhaled by smokers has an immediate effect on the system. As well as having a pleasantly narcotic effect, it causes the heart rate to accelerate rapidly. It seems that adrenalin is released by nicotine, and the sympathetic nervous system also releases an excess of epinephrine and norepinephrine which hastens the blood clotting process and damages the arterial walls. Thus nicotine raises the heart rate, increases blood pressure, and can cause a constriction of the arteries. It has been found that five smoke inhalations a minute can increase the heart rate by about fifteen beats per minute, thus increasing the amount of blood pumped by the heart and raising blood pressure. A single drop of nicotine injected into the blood stream direct would be fatal.

But it is not only nicotine which adversely affects the working of the heart. Carbon monoxide is inhaled as a by-product of combustion. We talk about carbon monoxide poisoning, and, indeed, the exhaust fumes from a car are often used as a means of pleasant suicide. The relaxation derived from smoking may be due to the carbon monoxide inhaled. But this gas combines with the red blood cells, thus depriving them of oxygen. At one and the same time then, cigarette smoking stimulates the heart to work harder and also deprives the heart of the oxygen its increased rate needs.

Smoking and other diseases

The relationship between smoking and lung cancer is well known and much debated. All that can safely be said is that the evidence strongly suggests that those who do not smoke are many times less likely to get lung cancer than those who smoke. The incidence of bronchitis is heavier among smokers than among non-smokers. Non-smokers are less likely to take in impurities which will irritate the sensitive lining of the lungs. Emphysema, a lung ailment with no known cure, is more likely to be contracted if you smoke. In this condition the elasticity of the lung cells is lost so that air cannot be properly expelled.

But it is not only the direct ill-effects of smoking which cause concern. The risk to unborn babies if their mothers smoke during pregnancy is well established. The obvious fact that if parents smoke their children are more likely to do so means that parents are aiding and abetting the risk of fatal disease in their own children.

Let us now spend some time on being more positive. Everybody knows that smoking, of whatever sort, is bad for their health. Let us see what *not* smoking does.

Benefits of not smoking

1 If you smoke a pack of cigarettes a day you will spend approximately £6.20 per week on cigarettes. This is about £322 per year. In a lifetime of smoking, assuming the habit has not killed you very prematurely, you will have spent about £12,900 on tobacco at the present rate. If you smoke forty cigarettes a day that is about £25,000 – or the price of a reasonable house. Non-smokers save money.

2 Your food will taste better and your appetite will improve.

3 Your physical efficiency, whether it is in running for a bus, getting rid of the smoker's cough, or lessening the changes of heart disease, will increase.

4 The risk of lung cancer would appear to be considerably lessened.

5 You will be more socially acceptable among groups of non-smokers. Certainly it is our belief that men and women whose clothes and hair stink

of tobacco are less likely to attract members of the opposite sex.

6 The feeling of having broken an addiction gives a sense of great achievement and confidence. Ironically, many people smoke to relieve stress, but abandoning the habit will so increase a person's confidence and independence, that he will be less likely to suffer from stress.

Breaking the habit

From the start let us not pretend that giving up smoking is easy. First of all you need to *want* to give up the habit, but because of the addictive nature of the 'weed' this is not easy. All we can say for sure, in the early stages, is that as far as the risk of contracting coronary or respiratory disease from smoking is concerned, at least *you* can do something positive to lessen the risk. Once you have stopped smoking, your heart, lungs and tissues will generally improve. Even if you have been an addict for many years, once you give up, your body will begin to improve, and the damage caused by smoking will gradually be repaired.

The initial feelings the smoker gets when he gives up the habit are unpleasant. The body has become used to its drug and suffers withdrawal symptoms when the drug is denied it. The sufferer has a 'nicotine fit'. He feels depressed and tense. He may feel more tired, gain weight, lose sleep, lose the ability to concentrate. He *will* suffer for a while, but as time passes the urge to light up will pass.

The cold turkey approach

We believe that the best way to stop smoking is just to stop. Try this strategy:

1 Decide on a day and time for having your last cigarette — or cigar or pipeful of tobacco. Preferably choose a day when your routine is already altered, or on a day, like a Sunday, when you can control the routine.

2 Throw away all pipes, cigars, cigarettes, matches and pipe-cleaners. Don't put them in a drawer in case of failure!

3 Hide your souvenir ash trays so that you are not reminded of smoking.

4 Announce to as many people as you can that you are giving up the habit — sticking to your word will give you added motivation.

5 Try to find others who will give up with you in order to strengthen your willpower.

6 When the craving becomes intolerable go for a walk, take a few deep breaths, do a job. All the time tell yourself 'I am strong enough to give up smoking'.

7 Set yourself rewards and punishments. If you succeed for the first few days treat yourself with the money saved to a meal out or a trip to the cinema. If you have backslid deny yourself a regular weekly pleasure, such as your game of golf or visit to the local cinema!

8 If you usually enjoy a smoke with a drink — as most smokers do — then cut out your visit to the pub for a while.

9 Many smoke after a meal. Get into the habit of going for a stroll after you have eaten, rather than remain sitting down while you smoke and drink your coffee.

10 Above all, think *positive*. Recite the reasons for giving up smoking. From the first day you will:
— be saving money
— be eating with more enjoyment
— be less wheezy and susceptible to coughs and colds
— have a more efficient cardio-vascular system
— be helping your children to grow up and stay healthier
— smell, look and feel better

11 When you are offered a cigarette get into the habit of saying, 'No thanks, I don't smoke'.

12 Remember that there will be times when the temptation to smoke is strong. You may feel and need something in the mouth or in your hand. Nibble a carrot or chew the end of a pencil. Invest in some worry beads. Do that long-delayed weeding or decorating. Avoid the temptation, often recommended, to chew gum.

13 Travel in non-smoking compartments and sit in 'no-smoking zones' of cinemas etc.

14 Open a 'piggy bank' account. If you are a twenty-a-day smoker you will be saving a pound every day. Over forty years, if you smoke as many cigarettes a day, at today's prices you will save over £25,000.

The cutting down approach

We think that this method is more difficult than the 'cold turkey' method, because you have not set yourself a positive goal; if you fail to reduce your intake one day, you may fool yourself into thinking that you will do better the following day, and so on. But if you feel that this is the only way for you, then see if the following suggestions help you:

1 Postpone the first cigarette of the day longer and longer.

2 Set up non-smoking zones at work and at home.

3 When you feel like a cigarette, delay the actual lighting of it for a few minutes. Try and eat something or do a job to prevent you from smoking.

4 Never smoke in bed if this is one of your habits.

5 Deny yourself the early morning cough! If you are starting a new regime of cutting down smoking with the eventual aim of cutting it out, it seems absurd to initiate each day with a cigarette.

6 Don't smoke before breakfast. Instead of breakfasting on a cup of coffee and a couple of cigarettes, treat yourself to food. Read what has been said in the diet section on the necessity for regular meals.

7 If you usually light up in the car or on the train to work, cut that habit out. On the train it is easy — go into a non-smoking compartment.

8 Get into the habit of leaving your office and home without cigarettes on you.

9 Don't smoke for an hour before a meal — get used to the fresh taste and smell of uncontaminated food.

10 Don't smoke during a meal. And if you must smoke after it, let it be only one cigarette. A two-foot cigar is not the same as single cigarette!

11 Limit yourself to one cigarette an hour maximum.

12 Don't smoke within an hour of going to bed. If you are a heavy smoker — i.e. one who smokes more than fifteen cigarettes a day — by bedtime you will be ceasing to enjoy it anyway. Your mouth and throat will be dry, your lungs coated with tar, such that the final cigarette will leave its harmful deposits in your lungs during sleep — a time when they can do their worst.

13 Record the number of cigarettes you smoke a day. Write down when, where, and if you can, why you had a cigarette at that particular time.

If you obey the above rules you will quickly reduce your consumption by half. By the end of the first week you should be increasing the intervals between each cigarette, such that eventually you break the habit altogether.

5 General benefits of exercise

Definition of aims

Before the full exercise programme is presented there is a number of important things to be said in order to help you more fully to understand what our joint aims are. It is important to remember that our concern is with the really unfit adult. And he or she may not yet be thirty years of age. We have defined this person as one who has a condition, such as high blood pressure or high triglyceride levels in the blood, conditions which he may be unaware of, but which, if untreated, greatly increase the risk of the person contracting some form of cardiac ailment or another. We have said that these conditions are unlikely to be detected in the normal High Street gymnasium. Thus the regimes suggested in this book will be of little relevance to the young man or woman who takes regular exercise, lives a relatively stress-free life, eats and sleeps regularly. But the regimes may assist these 'fit' young people to retain their healthy lifestyles.

Of course, you may not be able accurately to define your own state. The following five point classification of types may help you.

Super fit – the competitive athlete

Fit – the person who takes regular part in sport, e.g. the tenniser or golfer

Average – takes some exercise, but of an irregular nature

Unfit – takes no exercise at all

Really unfit – has a negative clinical condition, which perhaps he is unaware of, and which gives him a risky future

It is the last of these conditions that we are concerned with. And remember that 11-17 per cent of adults we have researched were unaware that anything was wrong with them. If you are over thirty years of age, live a predominately sedentary life, have an increasing work load, have a young family, eat large business meals, drink rather too much, take no exercise, are putting on weight, then it is almost certain that you are abusing your own body. For there is no doubt from our researches that you are

well on your way to coronary heart problems. If you smoke as well, and are constantly under stress, often feel acute anxiety and frustration, then not only are you becoming a less efficient physical machine, but you are becoming a more inefficient mental organism. You may well have found that you tire more easily, or that you have to work longer hours to achieve your working goals. Indeed, it is because we have discovered not only that inactivity, but also stress, plays an enormous part in cardiac illness, that many large corporations are now availing themselves of this system of treatment.

Remember all the time that we are dealing with four factors. Often you will find that the information given overlaps. This will help to remind you that a total change in your over-all attitude is desirable. Exercise, of whatever sort, by itself will not lift you from the really unfit class to the fit class, any more than will giving up smoking. By now we assume that you have decided that you are in our really unfit class or that you could be heading that way. We also assume that because you are reading this book you wish to do something about your condition. Let us further our discussion about exercise.

The first two things to be said are vital. The first is that we are dealing with protective exercise, with a system of training which is designed to minimize the risks to you of heart disease, or, if you have suffered from any type of cardiac malfunction, a system which will aid your rehabilitation. We are not concerned with competitive exercise. And we cannot repeat often enough that the average commercial gym knows next to nothing about protective exercise. They base their programmes on the type of training that fit, young athletes have done. Of course, it may be that after you have undergone the system outlined here you have promoted yourself to the fit class and wish to take up or resume some form of competitive sport. That is fine. But you must look elsewhere for guidance on training for competition. It we were to deal in competition, not only would we be asking you to work an already overworked

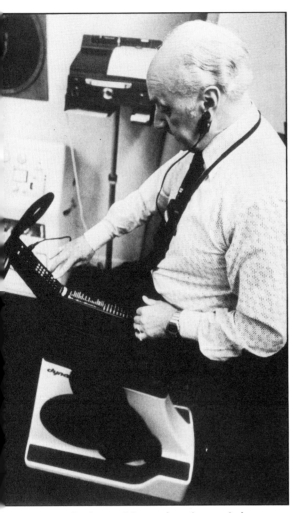

2 Computerized exercising and testing cycle by Jungeling

heart even harder, but in promoting in you a desire to do better than somebody else (and winning is the end of competition), we would be adding to your mental stress as well. It is immediately obvious when reading the chapter on stress how harmful excessive emotional arousal is to the functioning of the heart.

The second vital thing we wish to emphasize at the outset is that exercise that is exercise is exercise. It is, perhaps, the commonest fallacy, and sadly one sees it even in trained instructors, of the lay person to assume that the benefits gained from playing a game of squash are the same as those derived from soccer, yoga, jogging, cycling on a static cycle and swimming. Even with no technical knowledge of how the body works it is easy to see, after a few seconds' reflection, that the jogger is only

working his ankle, knee and hip joints; there is no way in which he is giving his upper body joints a workout. Similarly the yoga expert is getting very little heart/lung benefit from his contortions, though he may have greater peace of mind than the jogger and far greater all-round mobility.

We are concerned with exercising the whole physical man. We are concerned with general health, and remember, that playing tennis or riding a cycle ergometer, does not help you to alleviate stress or modify your diet. Just as exercise is not exercise is not exercise, so, too, is exercise not the only factor we must consider. So beware the fanatical squash player who forces you to be humiliated on his court by his assaults on your ego. Beware the commercial gym instructor who promises to make you Mr Universe in three weeks. Your concern is to reduce the stress (arousal) levels of your life, promote the efficient functioning of your heart and lungs, and to leave you a more relaxed, efficient person. From the last sentences you will deduce that as far as our protective programme is concerned we do not believe that if some exercise is good for you, more is necessarily better. As you will see later it is certainly possible and desirable in most cases to increase the amount of exercise you take. But equally, our researches, and those of others, have shown that as far as our aim of protection and rehabilitation is concerned, there is an optimum amount of exercise beyond which there is no measurable benefit to be gained. It was only after we discovered the minimum work load necessary to be done that measurable, hence beneficial, results could be made. Hence there is no one single activity which will give you the kind of benefits you need. And, indeed, it does not follow that if you took part in fifty different activities you would, by a process of elimination, have covered all the muscle groups, all the joints etc., that need to be exercised for you to have general health. The only certain process of elimination by such a method would be that of your elimination from this Earth! But be warned. We have found that people undergoing this comprehensive general programme have also been taking part in many other vigorous forms of exercise, thinking that they were doing themselves good. So, then, there is an initial problem of selecting your method of exercise. The average person is limited in making a selection because his experience of many forms of exercise is necessarily limited. Thus he or she may be led into a bad, dangerous form of exercise through ignorance. The system presented here is complete in itself, but as you become more efficient we will give advice on how to progress.

A final point to be made before discussing what happens when you do (or do not) exercise concerns another misconception. It is this. A fit person is not necessarily a healthy person. A healthy person is not necessarily fit. We may define health as freedom from disease. Fitness may be defined as the ability to reach a particular level of physical activity. It may be the level which allows you to cope with the demands of your daily environment. Any national coach will tell you that many world-breaking performances have been achieved by athletes who have had colds, sickness or been suffering from diarrhoea. Equally, we argue, any definition of health which limits itself to a physical implication, is a half-truth. A healthy mind is a necessary component of a healthy person. As Montaigne said, 'Man has a mind and a body, and we must not divide him.' Thus health implies a sense of physical and mental well-being. Fitness, a very specific concept, concerns the achievement of pre-determined goals. The fitness of an Olympic marathon runner is very different in concept from the levels of fitness our really unfit adult seeks to achieve. It is arguable, at the end of the day, that the achievement of his goal will make the really unfit adult a much healthier person than the marathon runner!

What happens when you take exercise

In this section we seek to explain in simple terms just how the body responds to physical exercise. We are not for the moment concerned with the physiological implications of psychological stress; these have already been dealt with in the chapters on stress.

The circulo-respiratory cycle

We all know that any form of mild exercise causes us to breathe more quickly. If we increase the intensity of the physical effort we may become breathless and be aware of the increased beating of our heart. Let us examine what happens when we are at rest. The heart's function, and it is a muscle, is to pump blood around the body. The blood which it pumps from the aorta has just been oxygenated by the lungs. Thus the blood which leaves the heart has had its supply of oxygen replenished. It is taking this oxygen to our muscles, which we can consider as a series of engines. The blood also takes fuel, in the form of chemical units of energy which have been converted from our food intake by the action of enzymes, to drive the engines. When this newly enriched blood has served its muscles, it is returned to the heart by the action of the muscles which work as a sort of peripheral circulatory system. If the

muscles are not accustomed to work they will work very inefficiently in helping to return this venous blood, as it is called, to the heart. The heart will, hence, have to beat faster to speed up the return, and will have less blood to squeeze out at its next contraction, hence weakening that contraction. The eventual result will be that if the heart has suddenly to respond to a large volume of venous blood it may well fail the test, with fatal consequences.

The venous blood, that is the blood which has just refuelled the muscles, returns to the heart via the lungs. As it passes throught the lungs an exchange of gases takes place; the so-called waste gases, like carbon dioxide, are expelled in the respired air, and the new supply of oxygen we have just breathed in re-oxygenates the blood. The above explanation is much simplified but from it it is easy to see why we puff and pant with exercise. Like any other engine, the muscles need fuel in order to function. If we drive the engines faster, or ask them to do heavier work, we use up more fuel. Oxygen and units of energy are the fuel supply. Thus, if we need more oxygen to complete our task we will get it only by breathing more heavily. If the engines are acting more vigorously in venous return, then our heart must contract and expand more quickly to push out the new arteriole blood, and, of course, to keep our supply of fuel strong. If the amount of fuel we demand is successfully supplied to the engine all is well. We are in a state known as 'homeostasis'. If, on the other hand, fuel supplies are insufficient to cope with the demands of the engine, we are gradually running into debt. And, indeed, the phrase 'oxygen debt' is used to describe this state which we have all experienced. At the end of a long climb up a hill we have all heard it said, perhaps by our grandmother, that she must sit down to get her breath back. And even top-class athletes who have excelled themselves are often very breathless at the end of a gruelling race. This business of getting the breath back is only another way of saying that they must continue to breathe heavily, i.e. take in supplies of oxygen, until they have paid their muscles the debt, and resumed the state of homeostasis. You are right to think that the muscles, unlike the internal combustion engine, can continue to function, for a while at least, with inadequate fuel supplies. The human body is a remarkable machine! But even it can only continue to function without oxygen, so-called 'anaerobically', for a limited period of time. This length of time is directly proportional to the over-all efficiency of the machine.

If the heart is in any way defective, or if the blood vessels themselves are in any way constricted, it is

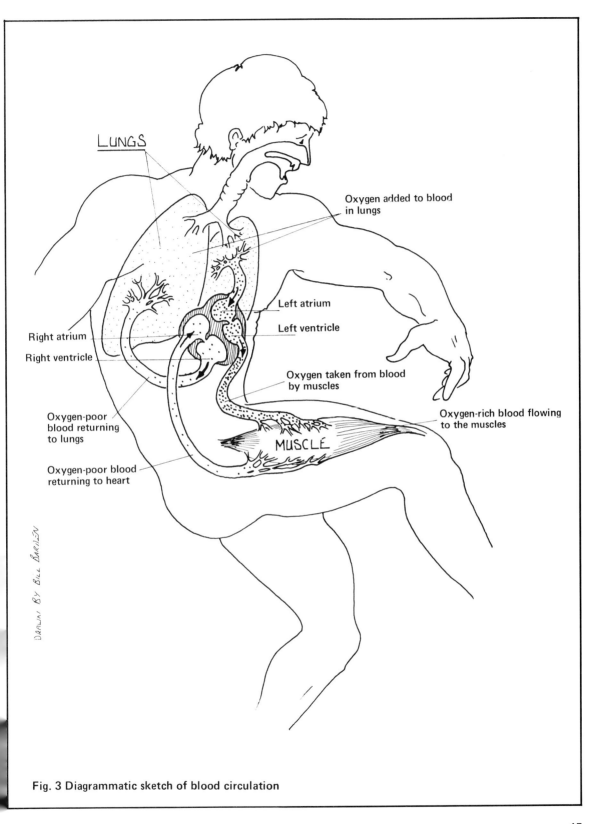

LUNGS

Oxygen added to blood
in lungs

Left atrium

Left ventricle

Right atrium

Right ventricle

Oxygen taken from blood
by muscles

Oxygen-poor
blood returning
to lungs

Oxygen-rich blood flowing
to the muscles

Oxygen-poor blood
returning to heart

MUSCLE

DRAWN BY BILL BARLEN

Fig. 3 Diagrammatic sketch of blood circulation

obvious that the engine will not function. It is not the object of this book to go into details of the intricacies of coronary heart disease, nor into the anatomy, physiology and metabolism of exercise. Suffice it to say that exercise appears to lessen the risk of coronary heart disease, and is a vital form of rehabilitative treatment. Cardiac arrest can simply be described as the sudden stoppage of blood flow. Total failure of flow in the heart causes death. The commonly known angina pectoris results from a narrowing of the coronary arteries and their inability to meet the heart's need for blood, particularly when the heart is responding to physical or emotional stress. The heart attack usually results from the narrowed arteries being completely blocked by a thrombus.

Exercise and breathing

We have just seen that muscles will not work unless they are fuelled. We have also seen that there are many ways in which the fuel supply can be interrupted — generally by some obstruction in the vessels (the pipelines in our analogy), but also by an inadequate pumping action on the part of the heart due to either too speedy an action or to an inefficient use of muscles in returning venous blood to the right-hand side of the heart. Let us look more closely at the processes involved in supplying this fuel.

The fuel, which is our energy supply, comes in two main forms. From our carbohydrate intake we get glucose in the blood, and we have fat as a second source of energy. The fat appears in the muscles as triglyceride, and in the blood as free fatty acids. Oxygen is required to act upon these fuel sources so that they may allow muscular contraction to occur. The harder we work, the more energy and oxygen we need. As a result the heart works harder and pushes more oxygenated blood to the muscles. The rate of breathing intensifies and all parts of the lung become more efficiently aerated. At the same time more blood 'saturates' the lungs than was the case when the body was at rest. Thus there is a greater volume of blood more efficiently oxygenated than was previously the case. Equally, as may be deduced, the removal of the waste gases, particularly carbon dioxide, is made more efficient.

Exercise, then, allows the lungs to play an important role not only in their ability to provide extra oxygen to help fuel the muscles, but also in preventing a build-up of waste gases.

Exercise and the muscles

Perhaps the simplest analogy one can draw between exercise and the muscles which we are able to control

concerns the chicken! We all love to chew a chicken leg because it is very meaty and, we notice that the leg is redder than the breast. These conditions occur because the chicken spends most of its time walking about in search of food. It, like us, walks because its muscles are fuelled by blood. Blood is red — hence the constantly 'blooded' leg muscles becomes red. As with the chicken, so too with our skeletal muscles. The trained athlete has large muscles. That is, there has been an increase in the size of muscle fibres. This implies that an untrained person has not allowed his fibres to achieve their full potential, or has allowed them to atrophy. Hence, any activity which requires a response from that set of muscles will be less efficient in the untrained person. Equally, the repetition of exercises through training seems to increase the skill level by which those exercises are performed, with a commensurate reduction in the effort required to perform the task. This explains why the coalman can shift tons of coal every day, but may well find himself exhausted if he is required to swim 25 metres or do any other infrequent physical task.

A final effect of exercise on our muscles is that they feel warmer; this increase in temperature seems to allow the muscles to respond to a call to action more quickly and efficiently. Athletes and dancers know the phenomenon as 'warming up'.

Thus with regular exercise our skeletal muscles increase in size, are more ready to respond to a call to action and assist in the efficient return of venous blood to the heart.

Exercise and the cardio-vascular system

The immediate effect of exercise on the cardio-vascular system is, as we have seen, to increase the muscle's need for more blood. During exercise the heart pumps out more blood than it does when at rest. Less blood goes to the skin — unless there is a crucial need for the body to lose heat — and to the organs in the viscera. Just as more blood is pumped out by the heart, so too, more blood is returned to the heart during exercise. And, of course, during physical activity the heart rate increases. The long-term effect of exercise on the cardio-vascular system will be dealt with in detail in the next chapter. In brief, though, the heart rate at rest, becomes slower. There is an increase in the amount of blood pumped out in unit time, the so-called stroke volume. The heart is able to do the same amount of work with less effort after a system of training. The heart also increases in weight as a result of exercise; this implies that the heart's efficiency increases.

Exercise and the coronary arteries

As has been stated, any malfunction of the pipelines (the arteries and veins which take blood from and to the heart, respectively) will result in a malfunction of the machine. Serious blockages may result in death. It has also been shown that exercise demands an increase in fuel supply, and that such an increase comes from the increased work of the heart. Because the blood travels along the arteries to the muscles, it follows that the efficiency of the blood to perform a physical task of increased severity rests not only upon the efficiency of the heart, but also upon the efficiency of the coronary arteries. In the case of patients with angina pectoris we have seen that this efficiency is found wanting. It is not possible to state categorically that exercise either increases the size of the coronary arteries or, where they are in some way blocked, that exercise assists in the development of vessels which lie alongside the constricted arteries. However, it is known that marathon runners have arteries which are two or three times larger than normal, and that it seems likely that exercise does allow alternate vessels to perform the function of blocked ones which lie alongside.

Conclusion

Exercise is beneficial to our cardio-vascular system and may help prevent heart disease. The complicated chemistry of exercise has not been gone into in great detail, but we shall have more to say about this in the following chapter. We have seen what happens when we take exercise. And we have seen that more exercise requires more fuel. The fuel is supplied from the bloodstream, and the efficiency of the supply depends upon the efficiency of our heart and lungs.

We can conclude that with exercise the heart becomes positively conditioned to pump out more blood, and that the heart beats less slowly when it is at rest than it did before its owner increased his physical efficiency. Finally, a 'trained' heart can do the same amount of work as an untrained one, but it will do the work with less effort. Let us now examine in more detail why these marvellous adaptations occur.

6 Outline of the exercise programme

The heart as an indicator

It was mentioned earlier that the normal High Street gymnasium could be a dangerous place for our really unfit adult to go to if he wished to improve his physical condition. We said this for two main reasons. One, that the system of exercise offered there was more often than not culled from competitive exercise programmes. Two, that there was no accurate way in which the work load, that is the amount of work you do, was initially calculated, nor was your progress – if any – monitored. Our system of exercise is entirely controlled by scientific criteria. We calculate exactly how much work you do, how often and for how long. We increase your work load according to measurable criteria. In order that you know all the time what you are doing and why, and know what this is doing for you, the various aspects of the physiology of exercise will now be explained in greater detail.

We have claimed that the complete system, not just the exercise programme, will help you to reduce the risk of getting heart disease or, if you have suffered from cardiac malfunction, will assist in your rehabilitation. So we are now going to concentrate on the heart.

We have seen that with exercise the heart becomes richer in oxygen, grows in size and in strength, and is capable of pumping more blood through the arteries. A trained heart can contract and expand more efficiently than an untrained one. That is, when it is working it pumps out blood more efficiently; when it is at rest it can take in a greater volume of blood. The more blood the heart can receive when it relaxes, the greater its efficiency will need to be in order to pump that volume of blood out. With exercise the heart attains this greater efficiency and hence feeds the muscles more effectively. They in their turn are more able to cope with the work demand put upon them. The muscles also do their bit by becoming more efficient in assisting the return of venous blood. Skeletal muscle like cardiac muscle alternately contracts and expands. An inefficient skeletal system means an automatic decrease in the efficiency of the heart; the heart will receive a smaller volume of blood, it will contract less forcibly to push this smaller volume through the aorta, and will be unable to cope with an unexpectedly high venous return. This may be the time to remind you of what happens to muscles which are not used. If you have ever broken a leg, you will know that all the time you are in plaster the muscles have been wasting away. The size of the unbroken leg is much larger than that of the broken leg. If the muscles are smaller they are less efficient. Just as unused skeletal muscle atrophies, so too do unused blood vessels close up. It is for this reason that doctors are in increasing numbers recommending that cardiac patients take up exercise; exercise strengthens, possibly increases the size and number of efficient vessels, so that a defective system can be by-passed. Certainly it is known that exercise lowers blood pressure, increases the efficiency of the heart and lungs and prevents the sticky blood platelets from becoming too severe a risk and gumming up vessels.

But how do we know what our heart is doing? 'Easy', we answer! 'We can feel it!' This is true. If we are very unfit and suddenly have to take violent exercise, within a few minutes or much less, we feel it pounding in our breasts. If we are about to be interviewed for a job or to propose to our girlfriends we feel it hammering away. In less extreme times we can discover how our heart is behaving by feeling our pulse. And it is because this system of training rests upon pulse rate control and a system of work loading, that so much time is spent here in discussing the heart.

But what about our pulse? The pulse tells us how often the heart is beating against the column of blood in our blood vessels. It is a wave initiated by the heart; it is not the heart beat itself. There is a time-lag between the contraction of the heart and the palpitation of the wave wherever you choose to feel it. Most of us are familiar with feeling the pulse at the wrist. Others may know how to feel it in the throat, or inside the thigh or at the head.

The rate of the pulse changes throughout the day.

If you have been asleep for a long time, its beat is slow. As the day progresses and you respond to the physical and emotional demands it brings the rate will increase. It will increase after you have eaten, when blood is being sent to the stomach to assist the digestive process. It increases with the artificial stimulation of nicotine, alcohol, coffee or other drugs. It increases with physical exercise and emotional anxiety. The pulse is a very accurate way of telling you all sorts of things. It will tell you whether you are hot or cold. It will let you know how the fuel supply is coping with the engine's demands. It will let you know whether you are excited or anxious. Now, all these things can be told in other ways, but as a single, unemotional guide to your physical and mental state it is a wonderful informant.

As far as we are concerned we want to know what it will tell us about our physical condition. The first thing it tells us is that we are alive — our heart is beating! If the pulse feels strong and regular when we are at rest we know that we are becoming fitter. If the artery at which we are feeling the pulse itself feels thick and elastic, again we know that we are fitter, for the reasons mentioned earlier. If, on the other hand, the pulse beats erratically, is hard to feel, 'flutters', or in any way deviates from the positive signs just mentioned, it is a sure bet that things are not as they should be. Of course, even the fit person's pulse can behave erratically if he is undergoing extremes of physical stress or mental anxiety. The difference between him and an unfit person is that his system is more capable of overcoming this extreme and of returning to normal more quickly. When you are at rest it is a fact that the lower your pulse rate, the more physically efficient you are. This is because the heart is taking more time to fill with blood, and hence fills more completely. The contraction which will pump this blood round the body will also be more efficient, there will be a greater supply of oxygen to the heart, and finally, of course, an improved coronary blood flow. It follows that our machine, our body, will function more efficiently as a result. A rapid, resting pulse rate generally indicates the reverse of all these things. The heart is given insufficient time to fill, oxygenation is less complete, coronary blood flow is impaired.

Exercise pushes up the pulse rate, but we learn very little about our condition by measuring this rate compared to the knowledge we gain from reading our resting rate. In general terms, incidentally, the resting pulse rate of men ranges from 72-76 beats a minute, and women from 80-84 beats a minute. The reason for this difference is not known. There are exceptions as always to this average. Some resting pulse rates in fit and healthy men have been recorded as high as 100 beats a minute, and as low as 35 beats a minute. If you have a high resting pulse rate, tachycardia as it is called, you should try to reduce it, for it implies that the heart is overworking; when you are at rest the muscles are not helping in the return of blood to the heart.

We have seen, then, that the lower our resting pulse rate the more efficient is our cardio-respiratory system. But how do we achieve a lowering of pulse rate? Ironically the way to lower our resting heart rate is to make the heart beat faster during periods of exercise. The increased demand of the heart to pump out blood results, as we have seen, in the strengthening of the heart wall and in the increased efficiency of the circulatory system. At rest, the trained heart uses this specific adaptation to good effect. It all has to do with economy. After regular exercise the heart's muscle fibres, just like the fibres of skeletal muscle, work more harmoniously together. They respond to the increased pressure of venous blood. After a time, according to the well-known SAID principle (Specific Adaptation to Imposed Demand), we may say the heart is used to operating at this more efficient rate. Thus when we are at rest it is still working with great efficiency. Each time it beats, it is pushing out a greater volume of blood than it did when we were unfit. This cardiac output is a crucial factor in determining whether or not we can cope with the demands of daily living or not. We need more blood when we are responding to physical or mental stress than when we are not. We measure the volume of blood by the amount which is pumped out per minute. This volume we call the stroke volume.

The only way we can increase stroke volume is by having our heart beat faster. If, though, our heart is a trained heart, and has all the positive attributes already mentioned, it will, under stress, be able safely to operate at a faster rate and, at rest, be able to pump more blood out in unit time, thus allowing us an economical and safe way of feeding the body. For this reason long-distance runners have a slow resting pulse rate; their training has so adapted the heart that it is used to pumping out maximum blood with each contraction when the body demands a high fuel intake; correspondingly, when they are at rest, the efficiency of the stroke volume is such that the heart need not beat very often to supply the body with its reduced demands for nourishment.

The elements of exercise

Now that we have explained what happens during exercise let us now consider a programme for the really unfit adult. Remember that we are concerned with protective exercise, and not with competitive exercise. Although it is true that all the adaptations we have discussed are applicable to both types of adult, it is all a matter of degree. We merely want to prevent cardiac disease and to be able to cope with our every-day environment, full as it is of mental strain as well as of physical demand. The competitive athlete under training seeks to tune his body to the extremes of performance. Generally he, or she, is training for a *specific* activity. Our aim is *general* fitness, as defined earlier.

Having decided on our aim, we must seek out methods of fulfilling it. In other words, we have to ask ourselves the question, 'What is the best way for me to develop and maintain a general exercise programme?' But even that question is not complete. We are all different people, with different occupations, different leisure interests, different standards of fitness. We want to know initially, particularly if we are very busy, how long we must exercise and at what rate. The answers to these questions are indeed surprising.

The programme may seem a low commitment to exercise on your part, but it will bring measurable benefits to you, whether you have suffered from heart disease or not. There are some instances where exercise will actually be harmful to you, but these instances relate solely to those who have a severe clinical condition. And in any case we advise no really unfit adult to embark upon a programme until he has been thoroughly examined by his doctor.

In deciding on the content of our programme, it is worth reiterating that any specific activity is of limited value as a way of achieving general fitness. We gave the example of jogging which, while being good for the heart and lungs and the joints of the lower body, does nothing for the upper body. Our programme exercises all the muscle groups and all the joints of the body and, at the same time, gives the heart and lungs the sort of work they need in order that they make the adaptations referred to earlier. The content of the programme is easy to remember. It is the three Ss — Strength, Stamina, Suppleness. (Most competitive athletes need to add the fourth and fifth factors, Speed and Skill, to their programmes.) We are to work our bodies to give them strength, stamina (what some call cardiovascular endurance), and suppleness (otherwise known as mobility). And we must decide on the Volume, Frequency and Intensity of the work. Before outlining the actual exercises in detail let us say something about each of these six key words so that you fully understand what you are doing.

Suppleness

Definition: The ability to turn, bend and twist with freedom and with grace.

We are concerned with every joint — the ankle, knee, hip, arm, shoulder, elbow, spine, fingers and toes. These joints should be flexed and extended over the full range of movement. As an example of full-range movement, if you stand erect with your hands by your sides and reach up and forward until your arms are vertically above your head, and then, aiming to brush your ears with your upper arms, you bring your arms downwards and sideways, you have completed the fullest possible circle of the shoulder joint.

With all these exercises we suggest that they are performed in a very specific way if you are going to get maximum benefit. Exercises administered by High Street gyms are often done sloppily; we would never give the command 'Arm circling backwards, begin!', because there is any number of ways to circle the arms. But there is only one way to do this shoulder mobilizing exercise to attain maximum benefit. But why do we need mobility? We know that lack of mobility may result in any number of the following:

— One shorter group of muscles. As explained earlier, muscles waste away when they are not used. If they have not been used through their full range they will atrophy. The result of this is inevitably a bad posture since the muscles are attached to the skeleton. If one set of muscles has been allowed to 'shorten' and, hence, limit the efficiency of one joint, then it is a safe bet that joints elsewhere are being worn away as a result of this distorted bony skeleton.

— Inefficient breathing. Our vital capacity — the amount of oxygen we can take in and use after one breath — depends in no small way on the ability we have to expand our chest. If the chest muscles and corresponding back and side muscles have been allowed to 'shorten', they will not be able to help us to expand our chest. Our heart/lung system will be less efficient than it was designed to be. And we must never forget that the body is designed to work in complete harmony. Shortened hamstrings or immobile lower limbs will affect the upper part of our body by pulling the skeleton downwards.

— An inability to respond to a sudden movement. If we are not used to exercising our joints through a full range, a sudden need to do so may well prove our downfall. We know that as we grow older we lose mobility — just think how 'rubbery' infants are compared to teenagers. When we become elderly not only do we continue to lose mobility but our bones become increasingly brittle. Many elderly people have falls which often result in a broken hip bone. This breakage, coupled with the shock of the accident, is frequently the immediate cause of their death. It is arguable that if they had been more mobile they would not have sustained the breakage. And *it is never too late to increase your own suppleness.*

Just as lack of mobility may result in any of the foregoing conditions, the possession of a supple body has the following advantages:

— It improves your appearance. You stand straighter, hold your head higher, walk more purposefully.
— It prevents many painful back and joint pains.
— It allows you to play your chosen sports more successfully and safely.
— It lets you respond to the sudden call to action in any situation with safety and confidence. We are talking, still, of protective suppleness. The suppleness of an Olympic gymnast has nothing to do with our aims.

You will notice when you read the instructions for the exercises that you don't need to do each exercise more than twelve times. We've seen people being required to do up to 100 repetitions in other programmes! Further you will notice that progress does not require you to speed up the movement; there should be no fast, jerky movements in the activity. You may find when you begin that you cannot move a joint through its full range. Always remember that progress lies in gentle attempts to stretch the muscles. Never forget that if you were able to flex and extend all your joints through their full range of movement, there would be no need for you to embark on this programme!

It cannot be emphasized enough that long, strong movements are the ones you should aim at. This is because muscles have a protective 'stretch reflex' which seeks to prevent you injuring yourself. For example, if you fling your arms vigorously sideways and backwards in a horizontal plane, you will find, particularly if you are round-shouldered, that there is a checking action at the end of the movement. The chest and shoulder muscles, having been vigorously stretched, suddenly contract to protect the shoulder joint. This sudden movement may result in torn muscle fibres or in injured joints. It is this extremity of movement which we wish to avoid. Similarly we would never recommend forceful straight-legged toe-touching as an exercise. Not only could you do damage to your joints by beating down to the floor, but often, the ability to touch your toes merely

indicates that you have long hamstrings — not that you have a mobile spine.

Indeed, it is often not known that there is an individual movement between each vertebra in the spine. Many of us are mobile in one part of the spine but not in another. The dorsal area of the spine (see fig. 4) is often mobile while the lumbar region is not. You can test whether or not you are mobile in the lumbar region in the following simple way. Stand with your back against a wall and your heels three inches away from the wall — to allow the back of your head and buttocks room. Your head should touch the wall and your arms be hanging loosely at your side. Pull the back of your neck close to the wall and hold that position. Pull in your stomach and try to touch the wall with the small of your back. If you *can* do it you have mobility in your lower back.

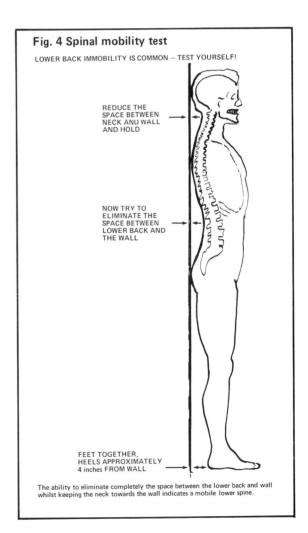

Fig. 4 Spinal mobility test

LOWER BACK IMMOBILITY IS COMMON — TEST YOURSELF!

REDUCE THE SPACE BETWEEN NECK AND WALL AND HOLD →

NOW TRY TO ELIMINATE THE SPACE BETWEEN LOWER BACK AND THE WALL →

FEET TOGETHER, HEELS APPROXIMATELY 4 inches FROM WALL →

The ability to eliminate completely the space between the lower back and wall whilst keeping the neck towards the wall indicates a mobile lower spine.

The last thing to be said about these suppleness exercises is that they are not designed to have any particular cardio-vascular effect. They will help you to achieve cardio-vascular efficiency but, of themselves, they are not cardio-vascular exercises. The five exercises selected for increasing mobility are the most basic of joint movements and are deliberately selected in order to avoid using complicated co-ordinating movements at this stage. Exercise 3 (page 65) replaces straight-leg toe touching, which can cause a great deal of unnecessary strain to the hamstrings and lower back — a point well worth noting both by exercisers and by teachers alike.

Spinal flexion and care

When spinal exercises are discussed, the first to mind is toe touching with straight legs. Unfortunately this is a badly understood exercise. Exercisers and quite often teachers are obsessed with how easy or how difficult it is for the exerciser to touch his or her toes. Two of the main objectives in straight leg toe touching are:

1 To increase the range of movment in forward flexion (bending) over the whole length of the spine.
2 To increase the range of hip flexion (bending at the hip) which is largely dependent on the range of movement of the muscles of the hip and rear of thigh (hamstrings).

Hyper flexion — dorsal spine. Note excessive flexion of the dorsal spine and complete lack of mobility of the lower back (lumbar region). Concentrating on merely touching the floor will only increase the mobility already present in the dorsal region and the hamstrings. Special key positions are necessary to ensure improvement in mobility of the whole spine. Results of course will also depend on the exerciser's age and other factors.

No spinal flexion. In this diagram we see a complete absence of spinal flexion. When witnessing someone with straight legs touching the floor with the palms of the hands we can be blind to the fact that this display of suppleness is accomplished by long hamstrings. Note that the angle between the body and thighs is quite acute and the back is flat. Toe touching in this manner will not improve spinal mobility (suppleness).

Spinal flexion. Here the exerciser is flexing both the spine and the hips; although ideal, it can be dangerous for the stiff, out-of-condition or older person. A competitive nature may drive one to overstretch the lower back muscles, ligaments can be damaged and the hamstring muscles pulled. The next diagram shows a much safer method of mobilizing the spine with a greater degree of safety, especially when really unfit. (See Exercise 3, page 65.)

Spinal flexion in safety. You can use the back of a chair to assist in keeping your balance. The left leg is lifted clear off the floor, this frees the pelvis, the supporting right leg is slightly bent to take the pull of the lower back and hamstrings. The lifting of the left leg is done simultaneously as the trunk and head bend towards over the hands. Exhale as you concentrate on bending the spine over its complete length. Repeat with the other leg.
NB The term 'long hamstrings' simply means long range of movement.

Strength

Definition: The ability to overcome a force through muscular effort.

You will see how inadequate the above definition is. The problem is that strength means so many different things in different contexts. Nowadays the strong man of the circus has been replaced by the Bionic Man of the television screen. We talk of a 'strong politician' or a 'strong character'. We may say that our coalman is 'strong' because of the tonnage of coal he manhandles daily — but as we saw earlier his strength rested upon the acquisition of skill. In physiological terms we may define maximal strength as 'the ability to move, ever so slightly, a load which the mover can only move once'. But even here we are in difficulties, for we can identify two methods of exerting muscular force.

The first relies upon our moving the muscle fibres — so-called isotonic contraction. Our ability to move a load through one repetition we would call maximal isotonic contraction. But equally we could exert maximum force against an immovable object; the joints would not move during the exertion, and we would call such an effort maximal isometric contraction. (Isotonic and isometric are terms which come from the Greek. *Iso* means 'equal', *tonic* we would define as 'stretched', perhaps, but with the implication of being returned to a starting position, and the movement repeated. *Metric* means 'length', i.e. we assume a position and maintain it without further movement.)

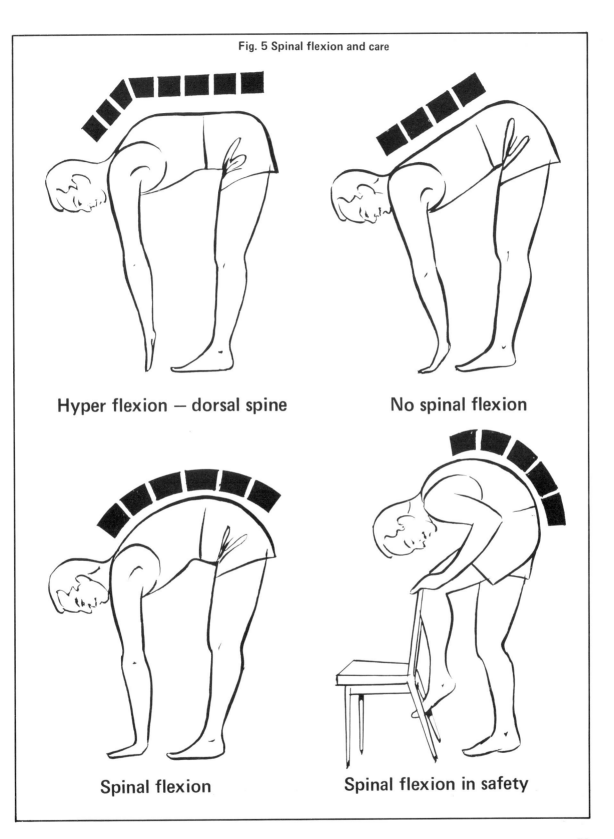

Fig. 5 Spinal flexion and care

Hyper flexion — dorsal spine

No spinal flexion

Spinal flexion

Spinal flexion in safety

But we are not concerned with extremes. Our principle is the SAFE one – Safe, Acceptable, Fitness-producing and Economic. As far as strength training is concerned, we wish to attain a state whereby we can fulfil our daily strength demands safely and competently. These demands vary, but the more we do a physical activity, like the coalman, the better we can perform that activity. Equally, the more we train all our muscle groups the more we will be able to cope with the unexpected.

At this point it is necessary to bring in our third S, Stamina. We can define stamina as the ability to withstand muscular fatigue. This implies that stamina, unlike strength, has a continuous implication. In short we can 'endure'. As far as strength is concerned we may only 'need' to do a movement once, in order to fulfil the demands of the definition. However, because we are not dealing with extremes in our programme, it will be easy to see that it is almost impossible to say where strength ends and stamina begins. For our purpose it is enough to know that any muscular effort which can be continued for only a few repetitions is strength training, and that any muscular effort which can be continued for considerably longer is endurance training. Thus the weight lifter who manages to press a very heavy weight once, is said, as far as that activity is concerned to be strong. The cyclist who can cycle for twenty-four hours non-stop we would say has stamina. But in both cases each man has something of the other quality in him. The weight lifter, to be able to train continually, must have local muscle endurance, and the cyclist, in order to be able to continue to cycle must have muscular strength. You see how relative all this is!

As far as we are concerned, we wish to build up local muscular strength and general muscular strength. We wish to increase local muscular endurance and general muscular endurance. We are not concerned with extremes of strength. We are aiming for a balance of strength and local endurance. The two go hand in hand. As we have already established, and, indeed as everybody knows, even a short-lived muscular effort, say moving a piece of furniture, causes the untrained person to puff and pant; so too does a longer-lasting, less 'strong' action cause us to puff and pant. In the first case we are doing a 'strong' activity, but because we are puffing and panting we are also doing cardio-vascular work; so too in the less 'strong' second activity, because we are puffing and panting we know we are doing cardio-vascular work, but we are also doing some strength work since we are overcoming resistance through physical effort.

It will by now be clear that those who play tennis, for example, are involved in stamina work rather than in strength work. For the closer you get to a resistance that limits your performance to a few repetitions, the closer you are to the idea of developing strength. But you will notice when you come to do the strength exercises, that in our training we are less concerned with five or six repetitions than with a greater number. We want lighter resistance, which is not only safer, but even more important, as well as improving our strength, it also has a beneficial cardio-vascular effect. (Remember our package deal of general fitness.) If the weight is correctly selected, and ours certainly is, then you are getting strength training *and* the weight is leaning towards local muscular endurance as well, and therefore you are getting increased cardio-vascular effect.

Stamina

Definition: The ability to withstand the onset of fatigue.

As already touched upon in the last section, improving our stamina, or endurance, depends to some extent upon the efficiency of our muscles. One of the reasons muscles tire is because of the build-up of waste chemicals within the muscles themselves. The most well-known is lactic acid. The more efficient our heart and lung system, the more will we be able to withstand the onset of fatigue. Similarly the more all the muscle fibres work in concert, the more efficient will they be in responding to a call to action. Muscles which are not used waste away. The important implication about all this is that you should take regular exercise all your life. There is certainly little point in taking a year's exercise and thinking that you can forego exercise for the following year or even longer! All the positive adaptations we discussed earlier which come about through regular practice apply as much to stamina training.

By now you will have realised that the heart and lungs are more intimately involved with stamina training than they are with suppleness or strength training. We hope also, though, that we have demonstrated that all three qualities go hand in hand, and that each is acquired more readily with the aid of the other. Indeed, this happens whether we like it or not! Our stamina exercises concentrate on the larger muscle groups. Sitting down and flexing and extending the fingers will have little cardio-vascular effect because the fingers are light and the muscles of the forearm which control them are small. (It is true that if you continue to flex and extend the fingers you will improve the stamina and local endurance of the forearm muscles, though!) Our stamina exercises work in the following ways:

— They use large muscle group activities, but our exercise sequence changes the groups.
— They are performed with some speed so that the pulse rate is raised.
— They are done continuously and without pause. Therefore the resistance chosen is sufficiently low so that the exercises can be continued for, say, ten minutes minimum.

This does not mean to say that each of our stamina exercises is continued for ten minutes! As has been previously explained, because of the nature of our programme the strength training, whether we use weights or not, does have a cardio-vascular effect. Our system requires that you *do not* have rest periods in between each activity, ideally. But, of course, in the very early stages you may need to have rests. It may be that the 'rest' is built into the pulse control for you at that particular time. Everything you do will be controlled by pulse rate, and not controlled on a trial-and-error basis — as is so much work controlled by novices and those who have no experience in training the really unfit adult.

In this regard we believe it is wrong to state that weight training has no cardio-vasuclar effect. It depends entirely on how the programme is devised. Our method of work loading and pulse rate control takes all the risk and uncertainty out of exercising, and has the advantage of exercising all the joints and muscles of the body. Consider the difference in result for the person who jogs for 20 minutes, and the person who spends 20 minutes improving the strength, stamina and suppleness of all his joints and muscles. There is no trial and error in our system. The pulse rate can be raised and lowered at will with the greatest accuracy, and we are not unduly straining one set of muscles and joints while totally ignoring another.

The pulse rate is raised and lowered during the whole schedule. We have peaks and troughs and a mean pulse rate. No research has been done to show that a consistently high pulse rate is better than one which goes up and down. All we *know* is that our system of peaks and troughs results in a lowering of blood pressure, and triglyceride levels, and in the improvement of recovery rate after exercise. Advocates of steady work, that is when the body does not fluctuate between high and low levels of heart rate, have yet to prove that theirs is the most efficient form of training. Indeed, research has shown that the heart gets more exercise with moderate fluctuations in pulse rate than without.

So, to recap, our strength training is a compromise between local endurance and real power. Our stamina work involves the larger muscle groups and a light resistance so that the work can be continued for at least ten minutes, thereby increasing the demand for oxygen and fuel. In protective exercise, all these requirements are governed by pulse rate control as explained in Chapter 7. We do not want the qualities of an Olympic athlete. Although, to see many fitness programmes for unfit adults, one would think that they were training for the Olympic Games! There is absolutely no need for the really unfit adult to train at pulse rates higher than 120 beats per minute in the early stages. Indeed, there is a point at which no measurable health benefit is gained by working at very high rates as in competitive sports.

Having decided that we must train for stamina, suppleness and strength, we must now examine the other three factors — volume, frequency and intensity.

Volume

It is important that you clearly establish in your mind what a 'correct' period of exercise is. We are concerned with protective and not with competitive exercise. The aims of both types of exercise are very different. Our national consciousness teaches us that 90 minutes of soccer, fifteen rounds of boxing, eighteen holes of golf, a school PE lesson of 45 minutes, are the norms. Thus you will find if you enrol at an evening class that you will be occupied in exercise for the local authority's statutory one hour! Some books advocate going from one level of training to a higher one. As far as our method and aims are concerned more exercise is not necessary. An exercise period of somewhere between 15 and 20 minutes is quite sufficient to fulfil our aims. If the system is right, and ours, which combines work loading with pulse rate control is, you will gain maximum benefit for yourself. You will not attain the highest levels of physical efficiency as seen in the super fit athlete — but, then, this is neither your nor our aim.

Frequency

Again, there are many misunderstandings — largely because most people who deal in exercise are trained in the atmosphere of competitive sport, or are trained to deal with the school or university population. We recommend that frequency of three times a week will enable you to develop physical protection of the sort we have described. It is true that if you train daily you will become fitter — but you do not need to do so for protective results.

Intensity

It is in this regard that most danger is seen. Because many of us, when we decide to re-embark on an exercise programme, tend to start from where we left off, perhaps ten or more years ago. We still feel a powerful competitive urge. We wish to keep up with our younger rivals — who may be professional as well as sporting rivals. All that this does is to increase our mental anxiety as well as put dangerous pressure on our physiological system.

Unlike the average gymnasium, our system regularly checks and monitors the rate at which you work. You are given, according to your current physical and emotional state, a working pulse rate which you elevate for 15 to 20 minutes. The degree of elevation is designed to give you protective fitness. If, after achieving this level of protective fitness, you decide that you wish to improve your competitive abilities, you will have to go elsewhere. What we will do is to reduce the risk factors in your state of health. We will help you to live a safer life by inculcating positive attitudes in your lifestyle. If, at the end of the programme, you have had success, and you will have had if you take our advice, then we will have done our job for you. More than that, you will be able to do your job in a more efficient, relaxed and economical way. If, thereafter, you wish to take up competitive sport again, that is fine. If you do not wish to, you merely have to continue our programme for the same positive benefits to be maintained.

But it is because your work rate is accurately monitored that our system works. Empirical observations, such as noticing the rate at which you are breathing, do not necessarily indicate pulse rate. There is no obvious correlation between heavy breathing and a high pulse rate. As we have already indicated, the pulse rate fluctuates for a variety of reasons:

— extremes of temperature
— physical exertion
— psychological stress
— illness
— after a large intake of food or alcohol.

7 Pulse rate control

In brief

We have been continually emphasizing that the success of our exercise programme depends upon our ability to measure, with considerable accuracy, the amount of work that is being done, and, also, to apply the results of our research to all ages and conditions of men, so that each individual has a personal programme to suit his or her needs. We need to be able to do this because, unlike the ordinary gymnasium, we are primarily concerned with the really unfit adult. Our business is protective, not competitive exercise.

The two factors which determine the exercise programme are work loading and pulse rate control. As its name implies, work loading concerns the amount of work to be achieved during an exercise schedule. Any work will increase the pulse rate. Therefore, we need to be able to control the pulse rate to ensure that the exerciser is not working at dangerously high levels, or, for that matter, at ineffectively low levels. Thus we cannot separate work load from pulse rate. The key word, though, is 'control'. And it is certainly the case that empirical observations of pulse rate are useless for our purposes. It is not possible, for a variety of reasons, accurately to assess the amount of work the heart is doing by placing your hand on your heart or by 'feeling' how heavily you are breathing. Different people have different heart rates anyway, and a high pulse rate need not be caused only by physical effort. It is worth explaining the principles of pulse rate control in greater detail.

Pulse rate control

You know what the pulse rate is. You know how to raise or lower it. You know what happens to your heart during exercise. The chart (see fig 6) illustrates how to calculate your working pulse rate. In simple terms, though, this is what happens. We make the assumption, based upon available research data, that a top-class athlete, at the peak of efficiency, has a maximum working pulse rate of 220 beats per minute. In practice the younger athlete, in the twenty to twenty-five year age range, is unlikely to exceed 200 beats per minute in training — partly, of course,

because of his extremely efficient cardio-vascular system. For our really unfit adult we take the starting figure of 200. If you are just beginning the schedule and/or are a really unfit person, you have an additional handicap of 40. You subtract your age plus the 40 handicap from 200 to give you your working pulse rate.

Thus if you are thirty-five years of age, in Week 1 your rate will be:

200 - (40 + 35) = 200 - 75 = 125 beats per minute. This is the same for men as it is for women. There is no danger in exceeding this rate but there is no necessity to do so. If you are under forty years of age, your handicap is reduced by 10 beats per minute weekly. Thus in Week 2 the thirty-five year old will work at 200 - (30 + 35) = 135 beats per minute. By Week 5 he will be working with no handicap at all, but will be merely substracting his age from 200.

This method of reducing the handicap week by week varies according to the age of the person. If he or she is fifty years old, then the handicap would be reduced by, say, 5 beats per minute per week. The exact reduction depends upon the individual. We are talking generally, but our researches have shown that there is remarkable accuracy even in this general formula.

Even with training, however, we recommend that the older individual retains some form of handicap. Even our fifty year old many well retain a handicap of 5-15 beats per minute — working, though he is, three times a week on our exercise programme. The fifty to sixty-five year olds, and the more elderly, may retain an even higher handicap. There is absolutely no need for you to work at a higher level. Remember, too, that compared with our super fit athlete our real handicap is not 40, but 60 beats per minute, for he would, by our method, be subtracting his age from 220. Don't be put off by the sayings of experienced coaches who state that there is no training effect to be gained unless the heart is working at 150-170 beats per minute. This is only true of competitive athletes, not of the really unfit adult who gets training effects from pulse rates between 110-120 beats per minute. Particularly is this true of cardiac patients.

You may be more easily persuaded of the efficacy of your method if you apply what has already been said to the effect of exercise on the heart to this new information. For, as well as reducing the handicap because the heart and lungs are becoming more efficient, you are having to work harder to maintain this new, and higher, pulse rate. This is a two-fold benefit. You have increased cardio-vascular efficiency, which, you will remember, manifests itself by reducing your resting pulse rate, hence you will have to do significantly more work to attain your new levels. The important relationship is between your starting rate and the eventual maximum working rate after training. Training at very high rates, *per se*, tells you nothing, except that you may, as a really unfit adult, be doing dangerous things.

Do not fall into the temptation of thinking that if 125 beats per minute is good for you, then 165 must be better! Remember what the pulse rate indicates. It tells you the frequency with which the heart beats. The faster it is beating the less time does it have to fill up. If it takes in less blood during a relaxation it will have less to pump out. This has a two-fold consequence. First, there is less fuel and oxygen going to the muscles. Second, the heart will have a smaller volume of blood to push against when it contracts. So, not only may the muscles be starved of nutrients, but also the heart will not receive adequate 'conditioning', because it does not have to exert itself against a large force when it contracts. At rates of 170-180 beats per minute this effect is experienced. And whilst it is true that the faster the

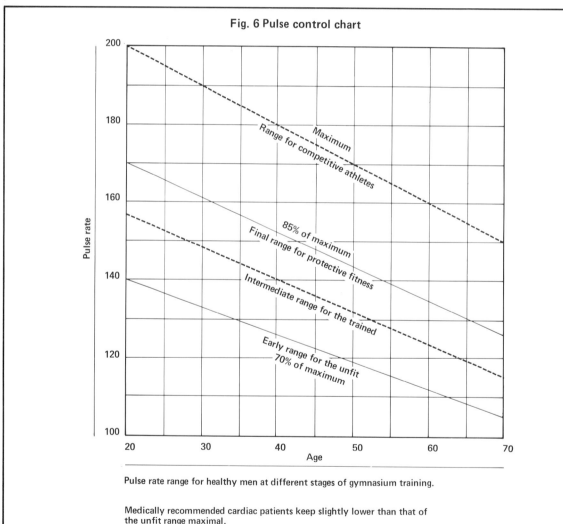

Fig. 6 Pulse control chart

Pulse rate range for healthy men at different stages of gymnasium training.

Medically recommended cardiac patients keep slightly lower than that of the unfit range maximal.

heart beats the greater will be the volume of blood pumped out, we have already seen that we are concerned with stroke volume, rather than just cardiac output. Everything finally depends upon the efficiency of cardiac muscle anyway. It may be that at 120 beats per minute you are unable to increase stroke volume because your heart is in poor shape. Our concern is to strengthen gradually and in a controlled way the efficiency of your circulatory system in a protective way. We are not training you for competitive sport.

How to apply pulse rate control to the non-apparatus exercises

Unless you are extremely unfit at the beginning of the exercise schedule or have suffered from a heart condition, it is extremely unlikely that your pulse rate will come anywhere near your recommended maximum in the early stages. This does not matter in the least, for our over-riding concern is with protective exercise, and the non-apparatus schedules are to prepare you for the apparatus schedules later on. (In fact, though, you will attain and maintain a high level of protective exercise if you stick permanently with the non-apparatus work.) However, it is a good idea for you to get practice by taking your pulse early on, so that you will be able to work extremely accurately later when you come to combine pulse control with the Murray Work Loading System. You will soon learn, for example, that the larger muscle groups will raise your pulse rate higher than will the smaller ones. We recommend that you take your pulse in the way described at the beginning of the schedule, and again at the end of it. It will certainly have risen if you have worked through the schedule without pause, but it may not have risen very much. This does not mean that you are doing no useful work.

Once you have got used to the schedules, you need only take your pulse rate after every three or four sessions. Even if the rate does not reach your recommended maximum at the end of a few weeks this does not mean that you are not working properly. Remember what we said earlier about the effect of exercise on the pulse rate. The more you work, the more efficiently you will work, provided you stick to the advice given and do not overdo it. If your heart and lungs are working more efficienctly then you will have to exert considerably more effort to raise your pulse rate. If the jogging programme is going to be part of your schedule then pulse rate may be more helpful to you. (See from page 72 onwards.)

Obviously as you progress from schedule to schedule you will notice that you are doing more work, so your pulse rate will go up. You will soon be

3 Pulse taking at wrist

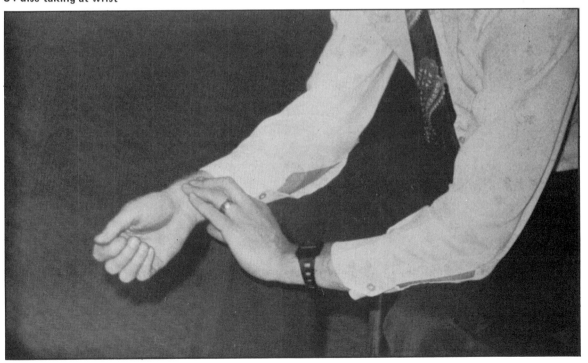

able to assess the rate at which you are working and will, hence, be spending less time in taking your pulse. The schedules are designed to be done without pause, so that you keep your heart rate up as much as possible for as long as possible, within the prescribed limits, and a cardio-vascular effect is being gained.

How to take your pulse

The success of this system of exercise depends upon your being able to take your pulse to determine your heart rate. The two easiest places at which the pulse can be taken are at the radial artery and at the carotid. We say below how the pulse can be palpitated at each spot, but would recommend that you learn to take the pulse at the wrist (radial artery).

The radial pulse

Take some form of exercise which will increase your heart rate — climb the stairs or run on the spot. Now feel your radial artery which lies at the front of the wrist at the base of the thumb. Place your finger tips near the base of the thumb. You will find there is a little groove in the wrist into which the tips of your fingers will fit. By pressing the tips lightly you should feel the radial pulse at the wrist. Don't worry too much if you don't feel it at first. Once you have felt it, count for ten seconds and multiply the result by six. If you count for any longer your body will gradually be recovering and your reading will be inaccurate. You may prefer to count for six seconds and add a nought to the result. But whichever method you use, remember to start your count with zero and not with one, or you will be a second out. In the early days it may help to count the pulse for 15 seconds, then multiply by four.

The carotid pulse

There is some advantage for exercise physiology in using the carotid artery in that you have one hand free to use a stopwatch. The carotid artery is the large artery in the neck which lies on either side of the Adam's apple. With a little practice you will soon be able to locate it. Place your fingertips on one side of the Adam's apple and press lightly. If you throw your head back you will force the arteries away from the front of the neck and make them more difficult to palpitate. If anything, you should press the head forward. Take the same ten or six, or 15 seconds' count. If you press too hard you will press on the carotid sinus and momentarily slow down the heart rate. Ideally you should take the pulse by this method with the aid of a stopwatch; only then will real accuracy be obtained.

8 The standard schedule without apparatus

General remarks

If you follow this schedule conscientiously you will be doing all you need in order to attain and maintain an acceptable level of protective fitness. The requirement is three sessions per week, each one lasting 15-20 minutes.

The five mobility exercises start each session, and do not progress. The strength and stamina exercises progress through four stages. However, it is possible that not everybody will want or need to progress to the fourth stage.

Summary of schedule:

STAGE 1 5 mobility exercises
Wall press-ups
Seated thigh raising
Chair squats

STAGE 2 5 mobility exercises
Table press-ups
Seated straight-leg lift
Squats without a chair
On the spot running

STAGE 3 5 mobility exercises
Chair press-ups
Floor sit-ups
Squat jumps
Bench stepping

STAGE 4 5 mobility exercises
Full floor press-ups
V sit-ups
Star jumps
Jogging, cycling or swimming

Posture: Strive for excellent spinal positions (fig. 4, page 57).

As for breathing, the following principles should be adhered to. Generally in exercise you inhale when the force is being applied, and exhale when it is being relaxed. When lifting, with the back extended and the sternum raised, inhale. In that position the chest cavity is being enlarged. *But* in some abdominal exercises, when the back is being rounded, you should exhale because the chest cavity is being made smaller.

5 MOBILITY EXERCISES

TO START EACH STAGE OF YOUR PROGRESSION

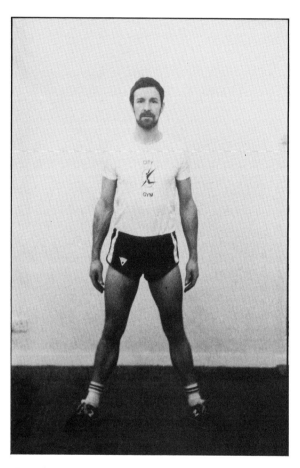

4a

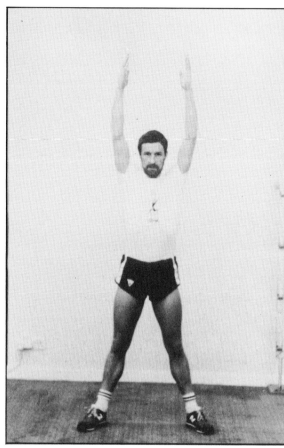

4b

1 Arm circling

Purpose: To mobilize the shoulder and chest region and to improve posture.

Starting position: Stand tall with feet wide astride, arms hanging loosely by the sides, trunk erect (*4a*).

Action: Raise both arms forward and upwards until the arms are vertically above the body and in line (*4b*). Keep the arms moving now downwards and backwards until they are level sideways with the shoulders (*4c*). Now relax the backward pulls and allow the arms to fall loosely by the sides of the thighs.

Breathing: Inhale as you reach up and lift the chest, and exhale when the arms are on the way sideways and downwards to the starting position.

Repetitions: 12

Comments: Do not force the stretching movement, and guard against arching the spine to compensate for lack of shoulder mobility. You should aim to brush your ears with the upper arms. Remember these are mobility exercises where *precise positions* are vital. (Such precise positions are not necessary where our main aim is cardio-vascular efficiency, i.e. jogging etc. Keep arms close to the body when they finish the downward sweep.

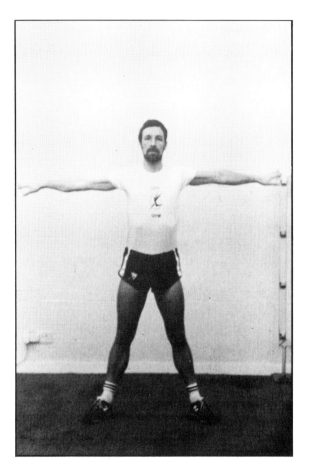

4c

2 Side bending

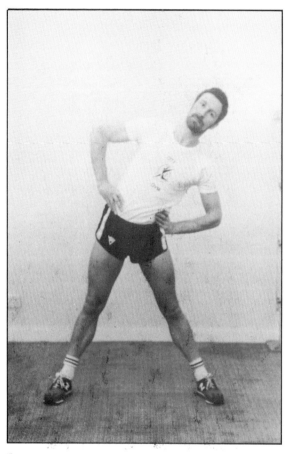

5a

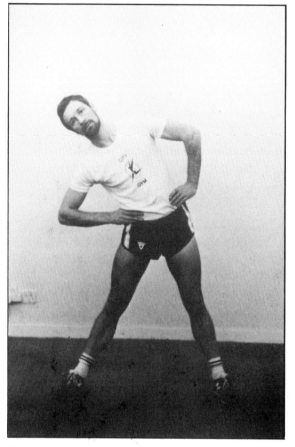

5b

Purpose: To mobilize the spine, and to improve the range of side bending.

Starting position: Stand with feet very wide apart, hands on hips.

Action: Bend first to left, keeping head at right angles to the shoulders (*5a*), then bend to the right without jerking (*5b*). Count 1 when you start to the left, 2 on your first bend to the right. Continue until you count 12 on the right, then stop.

Breathing: Breathe freely throughout.

Repetitions: 12 – 6 bends on each side.

Comments: Do not look down, but straight ahead even as you bend.

3 Trunk, knee and hip bending

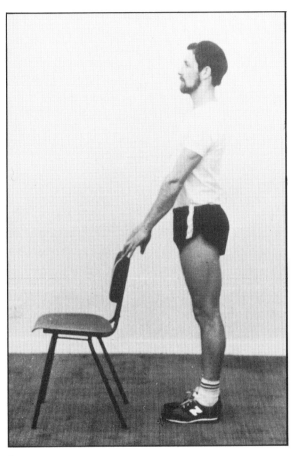

6a

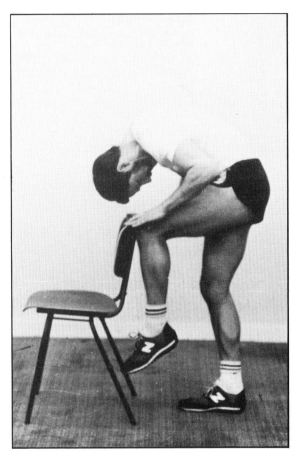

6b

Purpose: To mobilize the hip and spinal joints, and to give greater freedom in forward bending.

Starting position: Stand erect behind a chair with hands by your sides. Stand 18 inches from the chair, placing your hands on the back of it (6a).

Action: Transfer weight onto right leg. Raise left leg, but not as high as the hands. Lower the head towards the left knee (6b). Repeat for right leg once you have resumed starting position.

Breathing: Breathe out as you flex the trunk, breathe in as you return to the starting position.

Repetitions: 12

Comments: Do not let knees come near the hands. Do not look forward, but put chin on chest so that the neck, like the spine, is rounded. The supporting leg should not be stiff. Bend it slightly to reduce the pull on the back. Remember this is a hip/spine exercise, not a leg exercise. Stand tall between bends.

4 Head, arms and trunk rotating

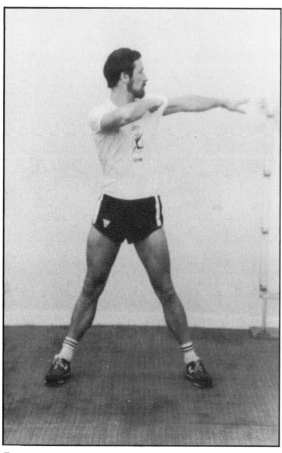

7a

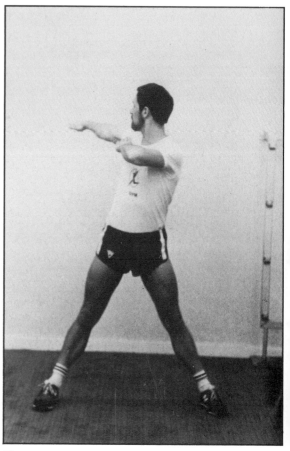

7b

Purpose: To mobilize the spinal joints, and to improve the ability to turn the trunk.

Starting position: Feet very wide apart, hands outstretched forwards in front of the shoulders.

Action: Rotate trunk to the left (7a). As left arm is going to the rear, look along it. At the same time slightly bend the right elbow so that it hugs the chest. The head, shoulders and arms should all be turned to the left. Then turn to the right side, bending the left elbow as it crosses the chest (7b). Aim to point directly behind you.

Breathing: Freely throughout.

Repetitions: 12

Comments: Keep pelvis and thighs still throughout the movement. If you are very mobile you may be able to rotate through 180 degrees. Do not swing or engage in a jerky throwing action. Keep hands in line with the shoulders. Stand tall throughout.

5 Alternate ankle reaching

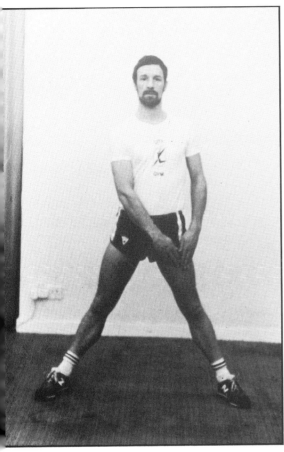

8a

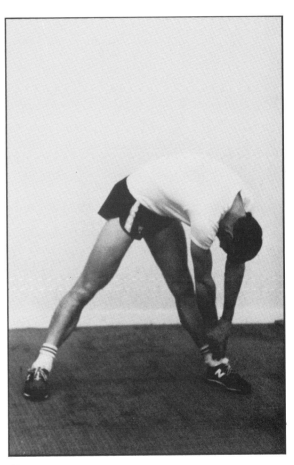

8b

Purpose: To improve the combined ability to turn, twist and bend the spine, and to stretch the hamstrings gently.

Starting position: Feet very wide apart, both palms against the front of the upper left thigh (*8a*).

Action: Let the weight of the trunk bend down and forward towards the left thigh, sliding the hands down the leg *towards* the left ankle (*8b*). Resume starting position by unrolling the body. Keep chin down, then the small of the back rises, then middle of the back, then the neck and then the head. As you come up let the hands fall apart to prove the arms are relaxed. (Remember these are relaxation as well as mobility exercises.)

Breathing: Exhale as the spine bends forward and inhale as you return to the starting position.

Repetitions: 12

Comments: *There is no target distance to achieve. If you have back trouble this exercise could be dangerous when you strain to touch the ankles or the floor.* Let gravity control the distance you go down. No attempt should be made to exceed a comfortable range of movement or to increase the speed. Stand tall between bends.

STRENGTH EXERCISES–Stage I

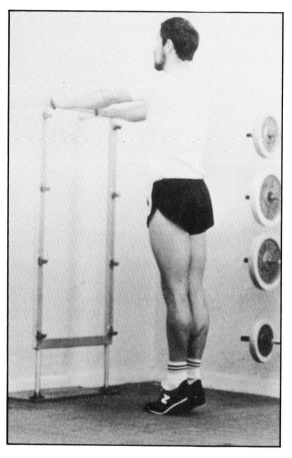

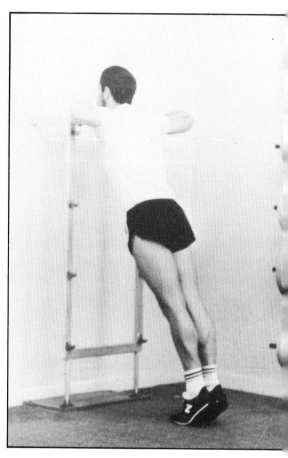

9a

9b

Wall press-ups

Purpose: To develop and strengthen arm, shoulder and chest muscles.

Starting position: Stand about 18 inches from a wall, with hands on the wall about 12 inches apart. Feet should be slightly apart (*9a*).

Action: Stand on your toes, then bend the arms until the chest and chin touch the wall (*9b*). Return to starting position by straightening arms.

Breathing: Inhale as you bend the arms, and exhale as you straighten them.

Repetitions: Begin with 8 repetitions, and gradually work up to 30 repetitions over a number of weeks.

Comments: Do the exercise rhythmically and comfortably. Don't progress too quickly.

2 Seated thigh–raising

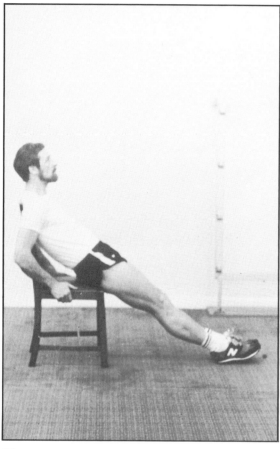

10a

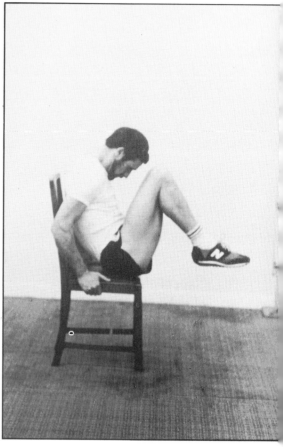

10b

Purpose: To strengthen abdominal muscles.

Starting position: Sit on the front edge of a straight-backed chair, or in an easy chair. Lean back and grip the sides of the chair for support (*10a*).

Action: Raise and bend knees up towards the chest, allowing the back to bend and permit the head to fall forward. Bring the fronts of the thighs up to squeeze gently against the body (*10b*). Repeat the movement.

Breathing: Exhale as you raise the knees and inhale as you lower.

Repetitions: Begin with 8 repetitions and work up to 30 over a number of weeks.

Comments: Don't sit right back in a straight-backed chair as you will inhibit movement. If you have weak abdominal muscles raise legs alternately. Progress at a comfortable rate.

3 Chair squats

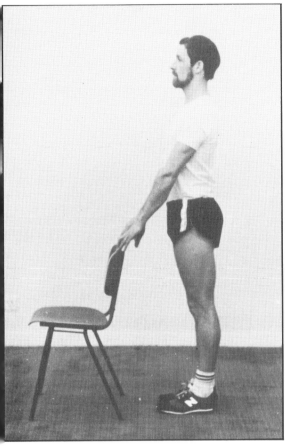

11a

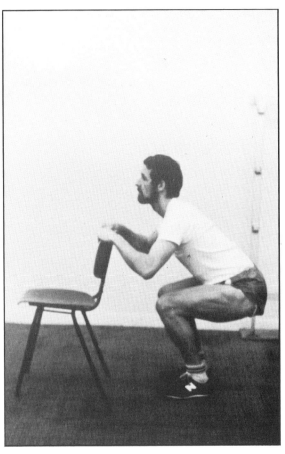

11b

Purpose: Mainly to strengthen the legs and hips.

Starting position: Stand 18 inches behind a chair, with your hands on the back (*11a*).

Action: Lower the body into a squat, keeping the feet flat on the floor (*11b*). Straighten both legs and come back into the upright. Try and raise onto your toes at the end of the movement.

Breathing: Breathe freely throughout.

Repetitions: Start with 8 and work up to 30 over a number of weeks.

Comments: Use a stout chair and grip it strongly. If your legs are weak keep your feet flat on the floor and pull strongly on the chair in the early stages. As with all the exercises, progress slowly.

Heart and lung exercise

Before suggesting various specific exercises which are designed mainly to improve your cardio-respiratory efficiency there are a number of points we would like to make by way of explanation.

The strength and suppleness exercises for all four stages of our non-apparatus programme have a good effect on the working of the heart and lungs. Earlier on we discussed why the pulse rate becomes higher with exercise, and how various good adaptations result from this. If you do the exercise programme here outlined without pause, you will find that your heart rate will increase during the schedule. In other words the strength, and the unchanging suppleness, exercises are of themselves good for the heart and lungs. If you can continue them without pause up to the maximum number of repetitions recommended you are improving your stamina. Thus, our exercises are of themselves *all* you need to do to maintain a protective level of fitness. And, they can all be done indoors at your leisure.

However, it is possible to improve your stamina even further, and at the same time to give variety to your programme by indulging in a number of additional activities. We suggest that you base your additional stamina exercises on the now very well-known activity of jogging.

We recommend controlled jogging as an excellent form of cardio-vascular exercise. It is also good for leg, hip and ankle muscles. Its obvious limitations have already been mentioned. However, jogging is not good for your health if you undertake it in a random way. Too many people now think that by donning a tracksuit and pounding round the streets of their local town for 45 minutes each evening they are doing themselves good. If they are in our 'risk' category and are running aimlessly like this, then they can soon develop respiratory troubles, probably joint and muscular problems as well, and will not only be unfit but unhealthy. We recommend the following:

It is essential to remember what was said earlier about pulse rate control when you read the following section. Fig. 7 will help you to understand the principles behind all progressive exercises as recommended here.

Imagine that you have completed the strength and suppleness schedules and are going on to do the stamina exercise. In the early stages we recommend that you walk four minutes from your home and four minutes back (Stage 1). If you are forty-five years of age, using our pulse rate formula you should aim to elevate your pulse by 200 - (40 + 45) = 115 beats per minute in Week 1. (It will be 125 beats

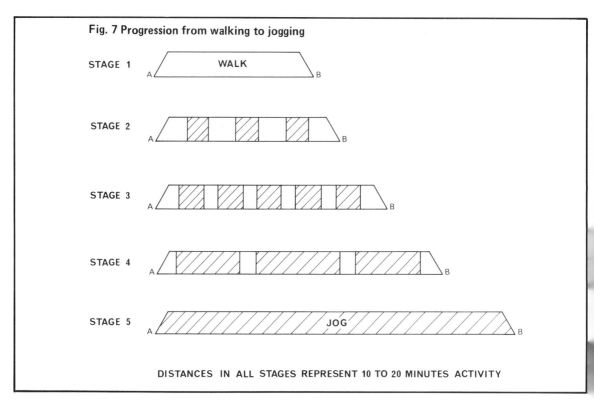

Fig. 7 Progression from walking to jogging

STAGE 1   A — WALK — B

STAGE 2   A — B

STAGE 3   A — B

STAGE 4   A — B

STAGE 5   A — JOG — B

DISTANCES IN ALL STAGES REPRESENT 10 TO 20 MINUTES ACTIVITY

per minute in Week 2 if you feel up to reducing your handicap by the full ten beats per minute.) If you have walked at the correct speed, and only two or three trials will enable you to do so, your pulse at the end of the walk should be 115 beats per minute. Soon you will find that you are having to walk faster to keep your pulse up. If you walk faster and still are aiming at an eight-minute round trip you will have to walk further to comply with the requirements of the task you have set yourself. Eventually you will have to walk so fast to keep your pulse rate up that you are jogging.

In the early stages you will find that you are, perhaps, not able to run continuously for eight minutes, or that to do so raises your pulse rate much higher than it should be, i.e. you will find that you need to alternate running and walking. We have shown you how to take your pulse and in the early stages we suggest you take it every minute or so. Soon you will be able to gauge with some accuracy whether or not it is significantly too high or too low.

Thus Stage 2 shows you how your progress will look. The shaded areas represent your jogging stage, and the unshaded areas your walking phase. We can call the walking phase a resting period, as the action of walking will reduce your pulse rate. Stage 3 shows the jogging periods becoming progressively longer and the walking shorter. Stage 4 shows that you are nearly jogging non-stop during the total eight minutes, and Stage 5 shows that you have eliminated the walking completely.

It is not easy to say with any accuracy how long this will take. The older person or the very overweight person may always have walking phases in his or her schedule. You may find that you cannot reduce your handicap each week. The sole criterion for you is pulse rate control. You know what your rate should be by simple calculation. Control your progress entirely on that basis.

If you are doing the full suppleness and strength programme there is no need to be out of your house for more than eight minutes. However, if you are not doing that programme then this progressive jogging can be done for 20 minutes. And there may be some of you who wish to do 20 minutes' progressive jogging on your 'rest' days. Eventually the younger person will have recaptured his youthful fitness and will wish to take part in other exercise. We strongly recommend swimming or cycling — but only in the controlled way just outlined. Finally it may well be that you will wish to take part in competitive sport — tennis or squash. This is fine. All we would say is that the older you become, the less competitive you need to be. Avoid the ego-trip! Try and find a partner whose attitude to sport coincides with your own. Someone who does not wish to win at all costs; preferably someone of the same standard as yourself. Use your head to protect your heart.

Thus our heart and lung exercise may well be progressive jogging. However, if this exercise is not possible we recommend an eight-minute walk.

STRENGTH EXERCISES–Stage 2

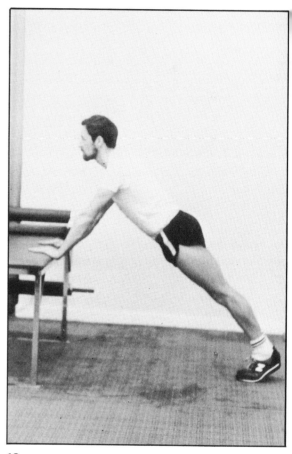

12a

I Table press–ups

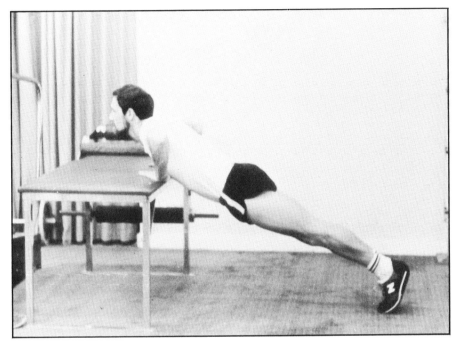

Purpose: To develop and strengthen chest, arm and shoulder muscles.

Starting position: Place both hands about shoulder-width apart on a secure table. Body should be straight and feet 10 inches apart. Have your feet far enough from the table so that when you bend your arms your chest touches the table edge (*12a*).

Action: Bend both arms until the chest touches the table (*12b*). Immediately straighten both arms and return to the starting position.

Breathing: Exhale as you bend the arms and inhale as you straighten them.

Repetitions: Start with 8 repetitions, and gradually increase to 30 over a number of weeks.

Comments: Progress slowly. Many of you, particularly the ladies, may not wish to progress after this stage on this exercise.

2 Seated straight-leg lift

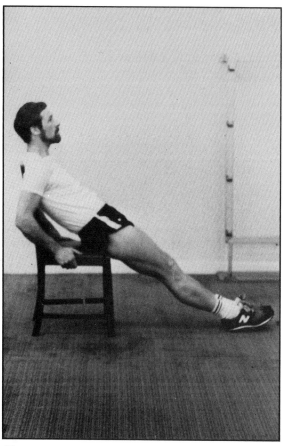

13a

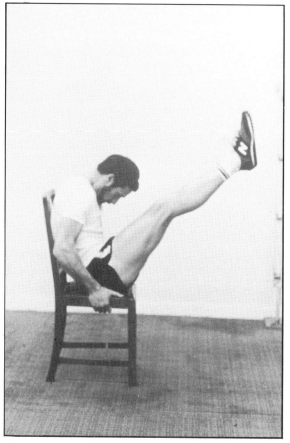

13b

Purpose: To strengthen the abdominal muscles.

Starting position: As for Stage 1 Exercise 2 (*13a*).

Action: Raise the legs off the floor until they are at right angles to the trunk (*13b*). Immediately lower them to the starting position.

Breathing: Exhale as you raise the legs, and inhale as you lower them.

Repetitions: Begin with 8 and work up to 30.

Comments: This is a very strong abdominal exercise. Care must be taken to do the exercise rhythmically and comfortably. In the early stages you may find that you are unable to raise the legs very high. Raise them only to a comfortable height before you progress.

3 Squats without a chair

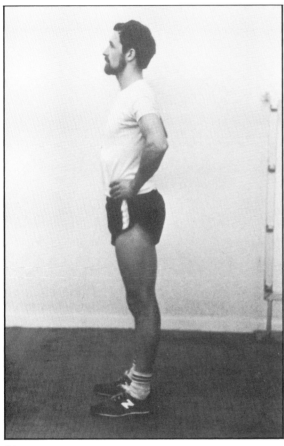

14a

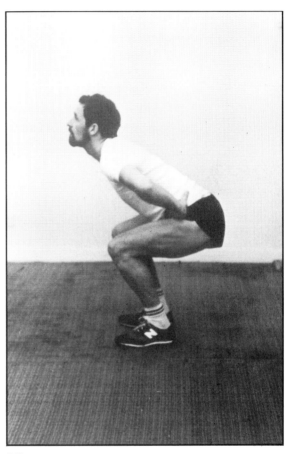

14b

Purpose: To exercise the leg muscles.

Starting position: Stand upright, feet slightly apart, with hands on hips (*14a*).

Action: Lower the body into a squat (*14b*), at the same time rise onto the toes. Resume the standing position on tiptoe. Repeat.

Breathing: Breathe freely throughout.

Repetitions: Start with 8 repetitons and work up to 30.

Comments: In the early stages you may find difficulty in keeping your balance. Experiment with different distances between the feet and do not lower your body too quickly. Look straight ahead.

4 Running on the spot

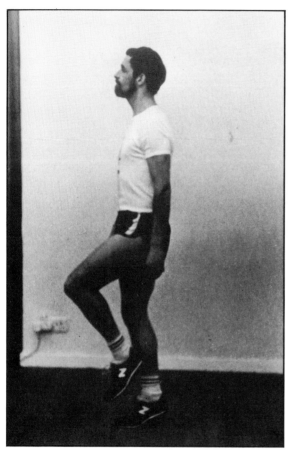

15

Purpose: To improve function of the heart and lungs (do this only if you are not doing the progressive jogging).

Starting position: Stand with arms loosely by the sides.

Action: Begin gently, making sure that you do not lift your knees high (*15*). As you become fitter raise the knees higher.

Breathing: Breathe freely.

Time: Start for only 30 seconds and build up to 5 or 6 minutes.

Comments: Use the pulse rate control to monitor your performance. Begin with the feet barely leaving the floor and progress to a higher stepping action. Remember you increase the work load by either lifting the feet higher or by increasing the duration of the exercise, or by both.

I Chair press-ups

Purpose: To exercise the chest, arm and shoulder muscles.

Starting position: Use two chairs, shoulder breadth apart. Place the palm of each hand on a chair. Keep the body straight with the toes of each foot on the floor (*16a*).

Action: Lower the body by bending the arms so that the chest comes to a position approaching the space between the chairs (*16b*). The really strong may allow the chest to dip between the chairs.

Breathing: Breathe freely throughout.

Repetitions: Start with 8 and work up to 25.

Comments: Use secure chairs. Don't try and lower the body too far in the early stages. Some people will not wish to progress to (or beyond) this stage.

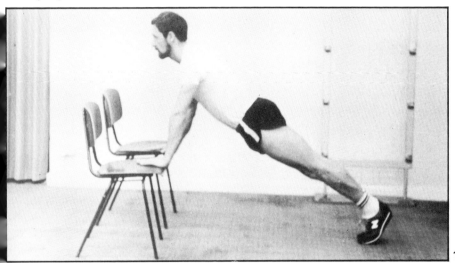

16a

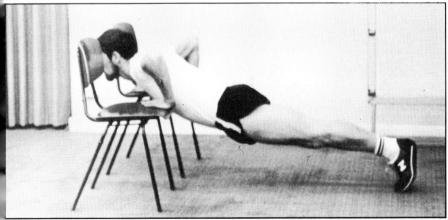

16b

2 Floor sit-ups

Purpose: To strengthen the abdominal muscles.

Starting position: Lie on your back, knees slightly bent with your hands over your head. Tuck your feet under a heavy chair or sofa (*17a*).

Action: Raise your body with your arms over your head into a sitting position. Lean forward and allow the hands to touch the ankles (*17b*). Resume the lying position.

Breathing: Exhale as you lift the body, and inhale when you lower.

Repetitions: Start with 8 and gradually progress to 30.

Comments: Do not attempt to touch your toes. If you find the exercise too hard in the early stages, bend your knees rather more. This reduces the pull on the lower back and hamstring.

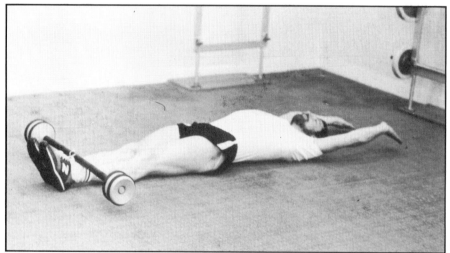

17a

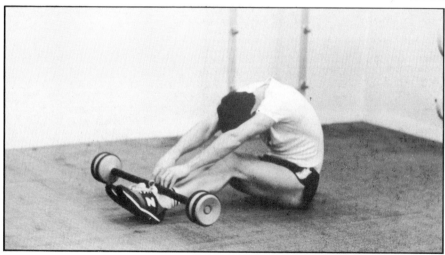

17b

3 Squat jumps

Purpose: To exercise the leg muscles.

Starting position: Stand upright, feet slightly apart, hands on hips.

Action: As in Stage 2 Exercise 3 (*18a*), except that you come *up* from the squat faster so that the feet leave the floor (*18b*). As you progress try and raise the feet higher.

Breathing: Breathe freely throughout.

Repetitions: Start with 8 and work up to a maximum of 24.

Comments: Do not try and jump too high in the early stages. As you land, go straight into the squat position. The height you jump depends on your fitness.

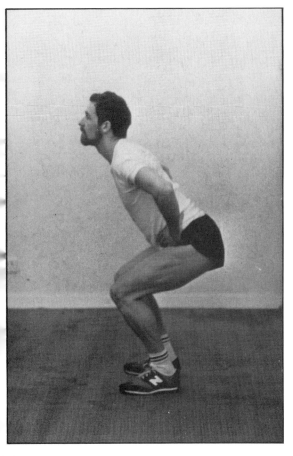

18a

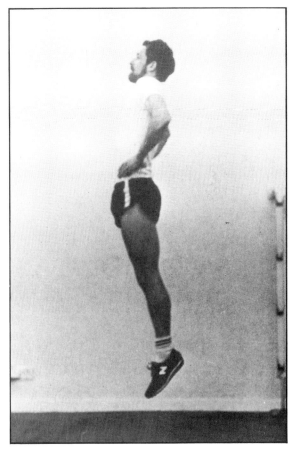

18b

4 Bench stepping

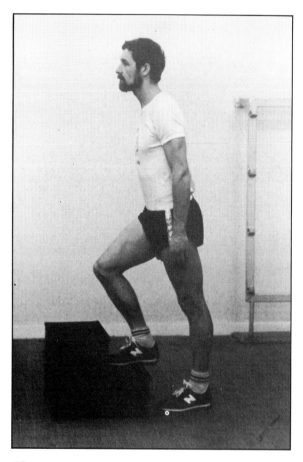

19a

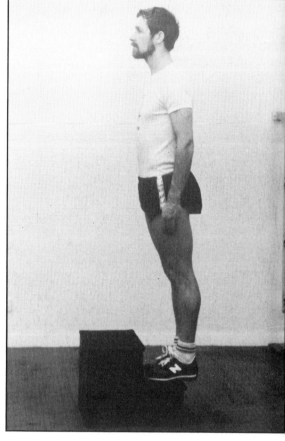

19b

Purpose: To exercise the muscles of the heart and lungs.

Starting position: Take a low box or stool and stand 12 inches from it. Place hands on hips or by your side.

Action: Step onto it with the left foot leading 15 times, and then with the right foot leading 15 times (*19a and b*).

Breathing: Breathe freely throughout.

Repetitions: Start with 30 and build up by one increase per session until you are doing 60, i.e. 30 with each foot.

Comments: Once you can do the maximum, increase the height of the bench or stool slightly. When you can do this, aim to repeat the exercise for 4 to 6 minutes without stopping. Use pulse rate control.

I Full floor press-ups

Purpose: To exercise the muscles of the chest, arms and shoulders.

Starting position: With body straight, place both hands flat on the floor. Fingers should point forwards or inwards and arms be about shoulder width apart (*20a*). Feet should be slightly apart, toes turned in and body resting on floor.

Action: Keep the body rigid and straighten both arms to lift the body off the floor (*20b*). Lower the body to starting position and repeat.

Breathing: Inhale as you press up, and exhale as you lower.

Repetitions: Start with 10 and work up to a maximum of 30.

Comments: Do not try and do too many in the early stages. You will find that if you have over-reached yourself the body will either sag or you will adopt an inverted V shape. Remember this is an arm exercise – a *push*-up.

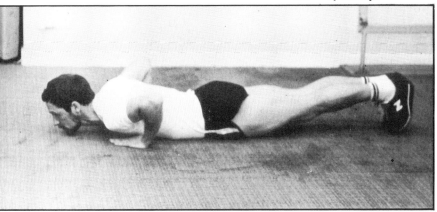

20a

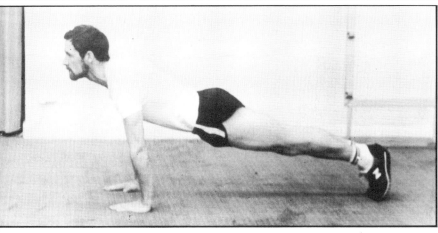

20b

2 V sit-ups

Purpose: To strengthen the abdominal muscles.

Starting position: Lie on your back, with your hands held behind your head and your heels on the edge of a chair (*21a*).

Action: Swing up to sitting position, allowing your knees to bend as you do so (*21b*). Return to starting position and repeat.

Breathing: Exhale as you sit up and inhale as you lower your body.

Repetitions: Start with 8 and gradually work up to 30.

Comments: Do not attempt to touch your knees with your nose! Do the movement rhythmically and progress gradually.

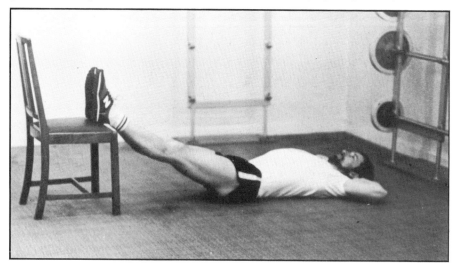

21a

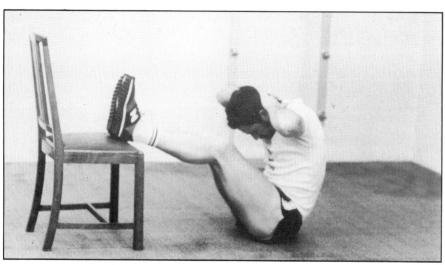

21b

3 Star jumps

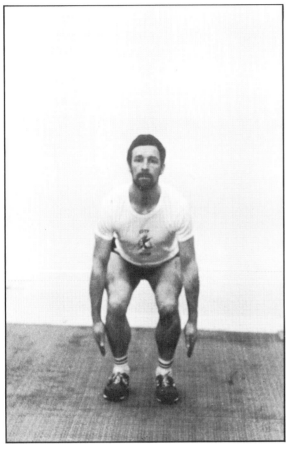

22a

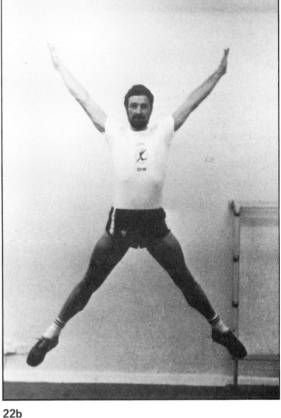

22b

Purpose: To strengthen the leg muscles.

Starting position: Start in the half-squat position with your hands straight out in front of you beside the knees. Feet should be a few inches apart (*22a*).

Action: Leap upwards, feet astride with arms raised in a star position above shoulder level (*22b*). Land on the toes and give at the knees to absorb the shock of landing.

Breathing: Breathe freely throughout.

Repetitions: Start at 6 and work up to 12.

Comments: Only a very few of you will be able to do this exercise. Do not attempt it if you do not wish to do so. If you are overweight or very unfit do not do it at all. (If you are very unfit and are attempting this exercise you are ignoring our progressive advice!!)

Jogging, cycling or swimming as a heart and lung exercise

By this stage you can safely jog, swim or cycle for 10 minutes without stopping. Regulate your exercise by pulse rate control — this will mean pauses for taking the pulse. As the weeks go by, you can increase your work by reducing your pulse handicap in the way already explained.

When should I progress from one stage to another?

You may have spent twenty years abusing your body! Do not expect to restore it to its former glory in twenty days. The schedules just described are progressively harder and are to be done at your own pace. It may be that you can do Stage 1 exercises easily at the first attempt. If that is so, and you are certain that you can do the maximum number of repetitions with comparative comfort — and within your pulse rate limit — then by all means progress. Go regularly from Stage 1 to Stage 2 to Stage 3 to Stage 4. Don't cut any corners. There are no short-cuts to fitness.

Some of you will not wish to progress beyond Stage 2. The older you are, the heavier you are, the more severe your clinical condition was, the less will you be able to do Stage 4 exercises. But because all the schedules have our mobility, strength and stamina ingredients you will, with all the stages, be guaranteeing a protective level of fitness. Experience only will tell you when to increase, say, the number of wall press-ups. Frequent taking of your pulse will inform you if you are working too hard or not hard enough. Aim at performing the schedules without pause — except when you think you need to take your pulse. Then, if the pulse is too high wait until it comes down. If it is too low, work harder. All that is written here is not Holy Writ. If there are fluctuations of ten beats either way in your pulse rate that is no cause for alarm. If you cannot initially do the minimum of eight repetitions — do six or four. We cannot prescribe a general programme of fitness which will to the nth degree suit all sorts and conditions of men and women. But if you use the schedules sensibly you will be amazed at the increased physical efficiency of your whole body.

9 The weight training schedule

Introduction

'Weight training' is a much misunderstood term. It is often confused with weight lifting. Weight training is a method of exercising the body which has much to recommend it. Weight lifting is a competitive sport in the course of which top class athletes attempt to lift the heaviest possible weight in a number of prescribed ways. There is no relationship between the two activities. Erase from your mind pictures of heavily muscled 'he-men', flexing their biceps while kicking sand into the face of an 8-stone weakling. Weight training is a conditioning activity. Weight lifting is a competitive sport.

Al Murray can claim to have introduced weight training to people all over the world. In his days as a National and Olympic Coach in weight lifting, he applied his methods of training weight lifters to the training of athletes in many other sports. After a long struggle against much sceptical opposition, weight training now forms the basis of training in many activities. It is used in track and field athletics, in ballet training, in swimming, boxing, cycling – in short, it is an essential part of the training of any competitive sportsman.

Our concern is with protective, not competitive exercise. And so, nowadays, weight training methods are applied successfully in protective exercise programmes. The heavy shoes used by those recovering from a broken leg and the resultant atrophy of leg muscles belong to the field of weight training. (Indeed, the Romans used weights on their wrists as a part of their boxing training, and on their ankles as part of their running training.) And just as the top-class athlete and the hospitalized patient can use weight training as part of their conditioning programme, so too can our really unfit adult avail himself of the many advantages of this activity. There may be some former 'ack-ack' gunners reading this book who will remember doing weight training with shells under the gaze of Al Murray in 1943! Many of his exercises are still being used today.

There are those who claim that weight training can have no beneficial cardio-vascular effect. As mentioned earlier, our schedule should ideally be done without pause. How, then, can the continuous raising of the pulse rate for 20 minutes or more at a rate which is specially calculated to suit *your* fitness needs, not have a cardio-vascular effect? Here is a list of some of the advantages weight training has over other forms of exercise training:

1 It can be used to good effect by all people. It helps the super fit, it helps the really unfit adult, and it helps all classes of people in between.

2 It can be adapted to all forms of physical movement, from ballet to badminton, from cricket to caber-tossing.

3 It can accurately control the exact amount of work being done – and remember the key to our weight training schedule is The Murray Work Loading System. It is always pleasant to be able accurately to chart one's progress.

4 It is a highly specific activity in two ways. First, because of the limitless range of poundage available, each person can have his own private schedule. (And his total work load has no relation to that of another person. If Mr Brown trains with a load of 6000 repounds in the course of a schedule, and Mr Smith with 4000 repounds, it does not necessarily mean that Mr Brown is healthier or fitter.) Second, because the exercises which are being done in the schedule are highly specific, there is a considerable amount of control being exercised on the muscle groups working. If the execution of the movement is correct, then it is known *precisely* which muscles are working. Hence, one can draw up a schedule and guarantee that all the muscle groups are being trained. It will easily be seen that jogging, for example, has severe limitations in this regard, for at best the ankle, knee and hip joints are being exercised, perhaps, over-exercised, whereas the other joints and muscle groups are being ignored.

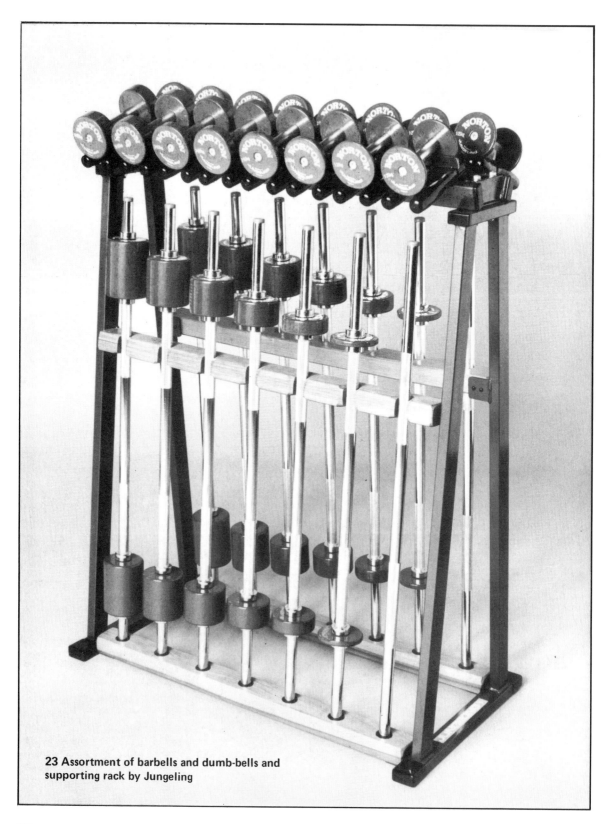

23 Assortment of barbells and dumb-bells and
supporting rack by Jungeling

As is well known, weight training can and does give, as we would more technically say, local endurance. It also gives general endurance as we have explained above. Jogging may give general endurance, and will give specific local endurance to the joints of the lower body. It will not allow the jogger, say, to saw logs all day, or to lift heavy parcels onto a lorry. Thus weight training caters for the whole body.

5 From what we have said in item 4, it follows that the correct application of weight training will not only increase over-all strength and stamina, but is an excellent way of improving our all-round suppleness. Twenty minutes of weight training is infinitely of more benefit to you than the equivalent amount of time spent jogging randomly. All these benefits accrue, of course, because of the accuracy with which The Murray Work Loading System can be calculated and applied.

6 Because the schedule contains both high repetition exercises to be performed by the large muscle groups, and lower repetition exercises to be performed by the smaller muscle groups, there is a system of peaks and troughs within the schedule. The high repetitions raise the pulse rate, the low repetitions lower the pulse rate. Because we are not working in the over-rated steady state way, but are alternating the intensity of the work load, not only can we keep going longer and hence improve our cardio-vascular efficiency, but we can also ensure that all our muscle groups are being given work, and that they are being given work appropriate to their capabilities. Fig.10 demonstrates how this physiological sequence functions.

7 It is necessary here to say that any individual can supply himself with the requisite barbells and dumb-bells at very little cost. We give information on this on pages 113-15.

Before we go on to explain the standard weight training programme the time has come to let you into the mysteries of The Murray Work Loading System.

The Murray Work Loading System

We have already explained that the unique feature of our exercise schedule is the combination of pulse rate control with The Murray Work Loading System. We have shown how the pulse rate control monitors the work done in the non-apparatus schedules, and how the practice gained in estimating the work done by different muscle groups is excellent experience for you in gauging your own progress and in learning

more about your own body. It is now time for us to talk in detail about this unique system for controlling the amount of work you do during the weight training programme. We have indicated earlier that empirical observations about the amount of work a person is doing are notoriously inaccurate in telling us anything about the state of the heart. We need a formula for calculating how much work a person should do, i.e. we must know at what rate to control his pulse, and we also need a practical system of work which assures us that this rate, as a mean pulse rate, is maintained.

Obviously we need these two ingredients in our programme to protect our subjects, particularly those who are recovering from a cardiac condition. We also need to be able to measure and grade the work load so that progress is achieved, safety maintained, and the long-term benefits realized. In what follows we discuss the work loading principle in detail, and illustrate it by the use of our weight training schedule and we give advice later on how to progress to a schedule with apparatus. We also give suggestions about how you can cheaply and quickly own your own apparatus if you so desire.

The system outlined here was devised electronically by a programme of research. Obviously it is impossible to wire every subject up to an ECG machine, or to take measurements by telemeter about what his heart is doing during the whole of an exercise schedule. However, this is precisely what we did before we drew conclusions which enabled us to formulate the work load formula.

We are concerned with three factors:

— the total number of repetitions in a workout

— the total amount of weight lifted in a workout

— the pulse rate from the start to the finish

We exclude the five suppleness exercises which start any schedule; even though they increase the heart rate slightly, which is, of course a good starting point anyway, work loading and pulse rate control really concern our strength and stamina exercises. The work loading system assists you to raise and lower your pulse rate at will during a full exercise schedule. It has already been explained how the larger muscle groups work to raise the pulse rate, and how the less strenuous work done by the smaller groups lowers the rate. A graph of the exercise schedule (see fig.10) shows a series of peaks and troughs as far as pulse rate is concerned. There is a measured physiological sequence which starts

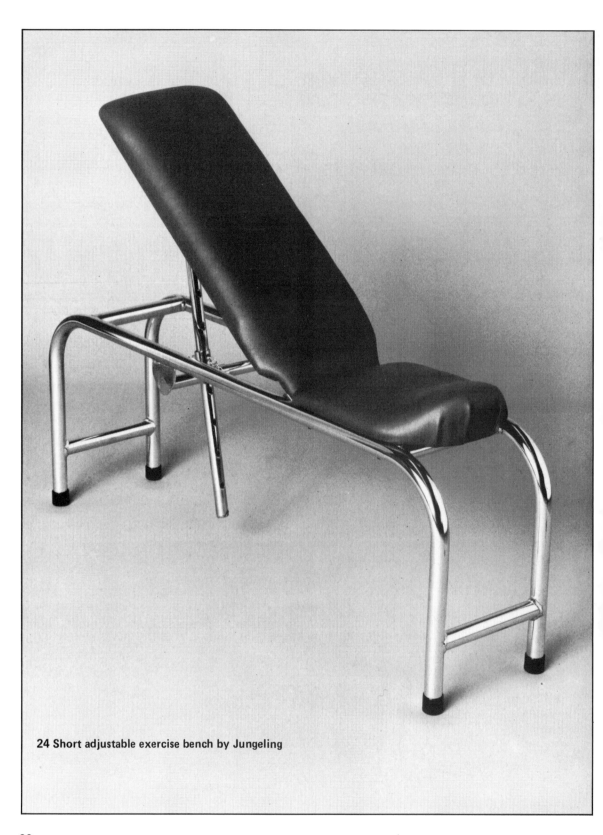

24 Short adjustable exercise bench by Jungeling

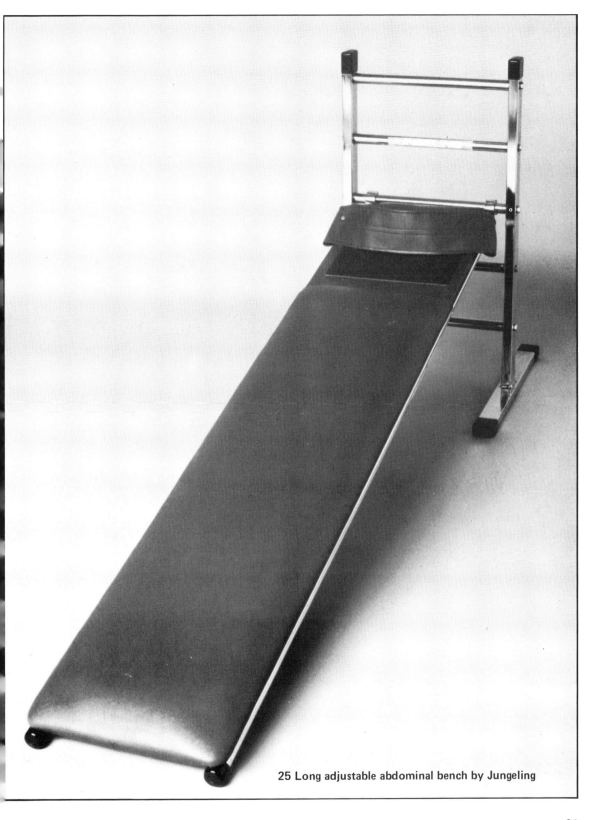

25 Long adjustable abdominal bench by Jungeling

at a relatively low level, increases to a maximum, and then tapers off as you come to the end of the workout.

We calculate the work load by writing down in a column the number of exercises and their names. In an adjacent column we write down the number of pounds which are going to be lifted in each exercise. Then, we total up the number of pounds and have a poundage total. In the third, and final, column, we write down the number of repetitions of each exercise and total them. Finally we take the time the whole schedule lasted, from Exercise 1 to 10.

For the sake of example let us assume that the total poundage for the ten exercises was 150 pounds, and that the total number of repetitions was also 150 for the whole schedule. Let us further assume that the total time taken to complete the schedule

was 18 minutes. To calculate our work load we multiply the poundage by the number of repetitions and divide the figure by the number of minutes. Thus, from our example, we have:

$$\frac{150 \times 150}{18} \qquad \text{repounds per minute}$$

(Repounds is a compound word formed from 're-petitions' and 'poundage'.) See chart on page 111 as a further example of how this works.

In addition we carefully select two stages in the schedule at which to take the pulse rate. In the example schedule (fig. 8) you will see that after Exercise 3, the press behind neck, and Exercise 8, the power clean, we take the pulse. We then divide these two pulse rates by two and arrive at a mean pulse rate. Thus, if after Exercise 3 the rate was

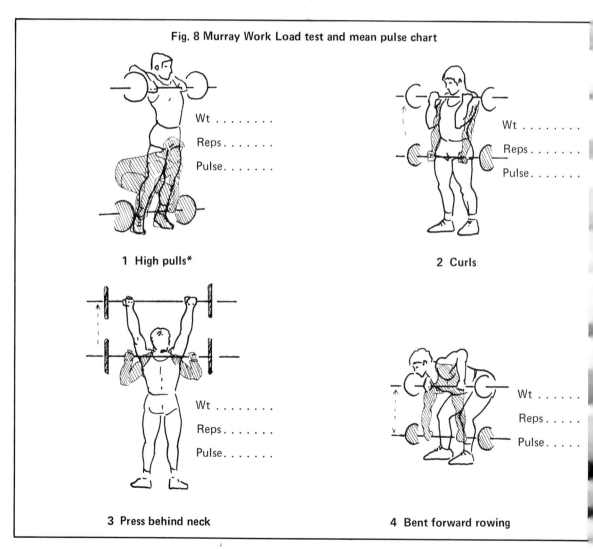

Fig. 8 Murray Work Load test and mean pulse chart

Wt . . . .
Reps . . . .
Pulse . . . .

1 High pulls*

Wt . . . .
Reps . . . .
Pulse . . . .

2 Curls

Wt . . . .
Reps . . . .
Pulse . . . .

3 Press behind neck

Wt . . . . . .
Reps . . . . .
Pulse . . . . .

4 Bent forward rowing

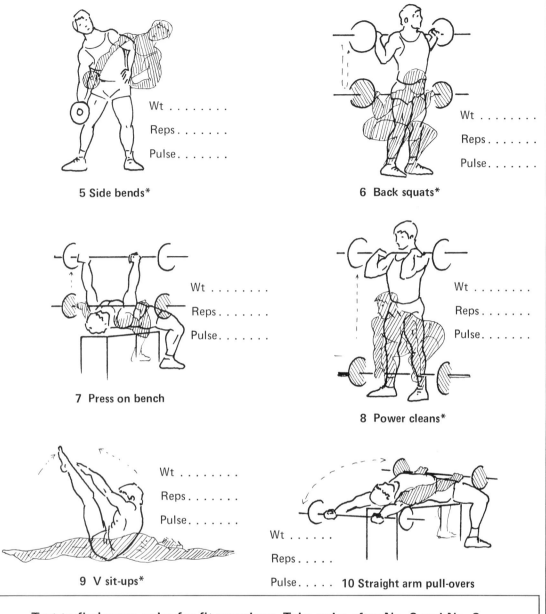

5 Side bends*

Wt . . . .
Reps . . . . . .
Pulse . . . . . .

6 Back squats*

Wt . . . .
Reps . . . . . .
Pulse . . . . . .

7 Press on bench

Wt . . . .
Reps . . . . . .
Pulse . . . . . .

8 Power cleans*

Wt . . . .
Reps . . . . . .
Pulse . . . . . .

9 V sit-ups*

Wt . . . .
Reps . . . . . .
Pulse . . . . . .

10 Straight arm pull-overs

Wt . . . . . .
Reps . . . . .
Pulse . . . . .

Test to find mean pulse for fit exercisers. Take pulse after No. 3 and No. 8, add both pulse rates, then divide by two.

Example: Pulse 1 + Pulse 2 ÷ Two = Mean pulse
(110   + 150)   ÷ 2   = 130

*HIGH REPETITIONS UP TO 30; ALL OTHERS 10 REPETITIONS.

PLEASE NOTE: ALL PROGRAMMES SHOULD BEGIN WITH THE FIVE MOBILITY EXERCISES

All illustrations are purely diagrammatic

Fig. 9 Exercise tempo for fitness

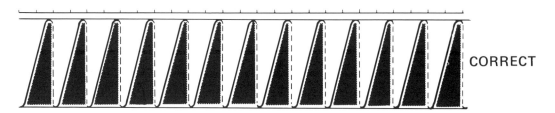

CORRECT

TIME OR EVEN REPETITION TEMPO DURING EXERCISE

Lift or Muscle Contraction
Lowering or Muscle Relaxation

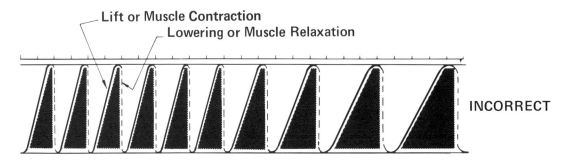

INCORRECT

TIME SHOWING CHANGE IN TEMPO TOWARDS END OF EXERCISE

WORK LOAD TOO HIGH   See note on B.P.

CHECK: 1 Weights
         2 Repetitions
         3 Tempo
        To reduce work load

The correct selection of the above three factors will permit the
Exerciser to complete the exercises scheduled without rests between
exercises or to exceed the prescribed pulse rate.

NOTE
The overall schedule Tempo must vary according to progress in
condition. The fitter the Exerciser the brisker the tempo throughout
the schedule.

A STANDARD TEMPO CANNOT BE LAID DOWN FOR ALL
INDIVIDUALS DUE TO THE VARIATIONS OF FITNESS LEVELS

B.P.
Blood pressure can be raised when tempo slows down and the
muscle contraction is held for a longer period of time due to high
intensity work.

110 beats per minute, and after Exercise 8 it was 140 beats per minute, their sum, 250, divided by two, gives a mean pulse rate of 125 beats per minute. Our electronic research validated beyond question the accuracy of this method of calculating work loading.

You will notice in fig. 8, the standard weight training programme, that there is a space beside each exercise for recording poundage, repetitions and pulse rate. You will also notice that some exercises have an asterisk beside them. The asterisked ones are those performed by the large muscle groups. We may start them doing 10 or 12 repetitions, and be doing eventually 30 or even 40 repetitions of them. This increase in repetitions will, of course, raise the pulse rate. The non-asterisked exercises are for the small muscle groups — the arm and shoulder exercises, for example, where we *keep* the number of repetitions low, and hence, lower the pulse rate. This is an example of the physiological sequence in action.

In fact, the work loading principle never changes. Pulse rate control does change as we have seen. Thus for our standard weight training programme if we do the five non-asterisked exercises for 12 repetitions each, and the five asterisked exercises for 30 repetitions each, and if we lift p pounds and take t minutes for the whole schedule to be completed, our repounds per minute are:

$$\frac{(5 \times 12) + (5 \times 30) \text{ repetitions} \times p \text{ poundage}}{t \text{ minutes}}$$

$$= \frac{210p}{t} \quad \text{repounds per minute}$$

This is all rather complicated, but you should be able to see that by calculating a mean pulse rate according to the principles of pulse rate control, and by applying this figure to the work loading method just outlined, the amount of work you do, and the control which you have over your programme, is very accurate.

As you progress you will need to alter your volume of work. This can be done in three ways:
- by working faster, thus reducing the time of the schedule and, hence, the figure by which you divide the product of repetitions and poundage
- by increasing the number of repetitions
- by increasing the poundage

In practice the exercises are started at a moderate speed. As time goes on the tempo is increased and/or the number of repetitions. The poundage is not increased until the maximum number of repetitions can be reached on the asterisked exercises. This is because the most efficient work is done at higher repetitions, and not at lower repetitions with heavier weights. You must not progress too quickly.

The arm and shoulder exercises, on our diagram Exercise 2, 3, 4, 7 and 10 will demand less oxygen than the other exercises. They are placed in the schedule to reduce the pulse rate where we so desire. The mean pulse rate comes in the middle of the sequence approximately. And we must also remember that in the schedule the cumulative effect of the pulse rate increases as the schedule progresses. If you look at fig. 10 both the peaks and troughs are getting higher. The mean pulse rate lies somewhere between the highest peak and the lowest trough.

The alternation of high pulse rates with low rates is, you will remember, so that you do not become too fatigued in any one area. Our aim is to complete the schedule non-stop, to gain maximum strength and stamina benefits, and, hence, maximum cardiovascular improvement. Thus we wish you to do all the exercises, of whatever sort, at an even tempo. Each muscular contraction should be followed by full relaxation. Our aim is contraction-relaxation, contraction-relaxation. We do not want contraction-contraction-contraction as may be the aim of the competitive athlete. It is known, furthermore, that isometric work — where the muscle fibres are held in a state of contraction — is dangerous for the individual with high blood pressure. This is because isometric contractions, particularly very heavy ones, make the muscle hard and force blood out of the arteries. This blood has to go elsewhere in the circulatory system, and will cause unnatural pressures there. Consider what happens when you stand on part of the circumference of an inflated car inner tube. Unless the tube bursts the displaced air appears elsewhere, causing distortion in the shape (see fig. 11).

You may find that despite accurate pulse rate control and work loading, despite having learned the correct tempo at which to work, your heart and lungs exceed the pulse rate set for you. If this happens, any or all of tempo, resistance and number of repetitions can, and should, be reduced. If you find that between exercises you have to rest, then your work load should be reduced. You will find that it takes a certain amount of trial and error to work at the optimum rate and with the correct loading. However, once you have been given a mean pulse rate and have worked through the whole schedule, recording the poundage, repetition and pulse rate for each exercise, you will be able to calculate with a large degree of accuracy your own schedule.

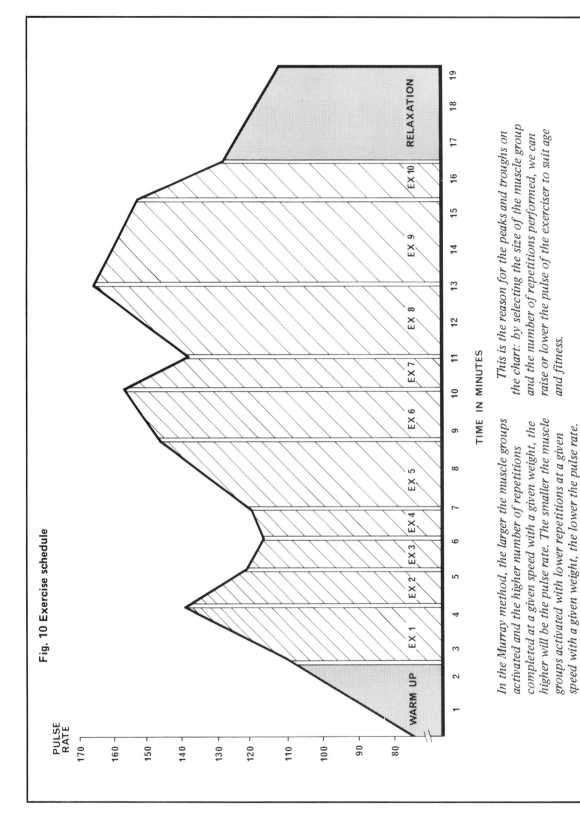

Fig. 10 Exercise schedule

In the Murray method, the larger the muscle groups activated and the higher number of repetitions completed at a given speed with a given weight, the higher will be the pulse rate. The smaller the muscle groups activated with lower repetitions at a given speed with a given weight, the lower the pulse rate.

This is the reason for the peaks and troughs on the chart: by selecting the size of the muscle group and the number of repetitions performed, we can raise or lower the pulse of the exerciser to suit age and fitness.

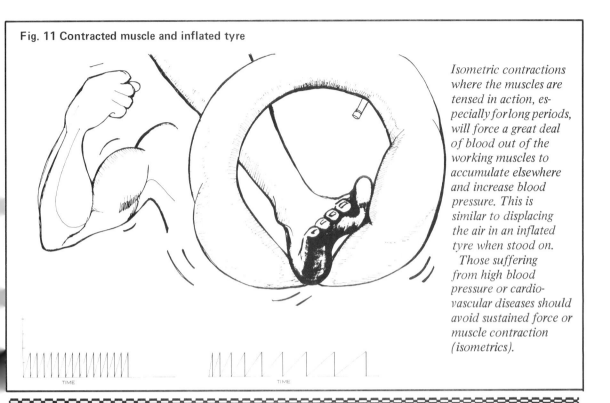

Fig. 11 Contracted muscle and inflated tyre

Isometric contractions where the muscles are tensed in action, especially for long periods, will force a great deal of blood out of the working muscles to accumulate elsewhere and increase blood pressure. This is similar to displacing the air in an inflated tyre when stood on.

Those suffering from high blood pressure or cardio-vascular diseases should avoid sustained force or muscle contraction (isometrics).

THE STANDARD WEIGHT TRAINING PROGRAMME

By the time you embark on this programme you will have completed successfully the non-apparatus schedules, and will, already, have improved your physical efficiency. Before starting this programme you must begin with the original five mobility exercises. Start with these during every training programme you undertake.

Five of the exercises have this symbol * next to them, and five do not. Those which do are the exercises which apply to the larger muscle groups, and your eventual aim is to do up to 30, or even, 40 repetitions of the movement. For all the other exercises you do a steady 10 repetitions. As you become more efficient you will raise the poundage rather than increase the repetitions. The asterisked exercises represent our peaks, the others our troughs.

Before you start the schedule you must know how to lift weights safely. The first thing that needs to be

said, then, is never attempt to lift a heavier weight than you can comfortably manage.

The correct way to pick the barbell up at the start of each relevant exercise is as follows. Place your feet under the barbell, hip-width apart. Place hands in overgrasp, shoulder-width apart, on the barbell and look straight ahead. Bend knees to about 90 degrees, have your back flat, not vertical, your arms straight but not rigid, and straighten your legs until the barbell is across your thighs. You will be in an appropriate 'attention' position. There are two basic grips. One is called 'overgrasp', the other 'under-grasp'. In overgrasp the bar is held so that your fingers are placed on top of the bar before you curl them round the bar. In undergrasp the fingers are placed under the bar before grasping it. In over-grasp the backs of your hands are uppermost, in undergrasp your palms face upwards.

===

I High chin pulls*

===

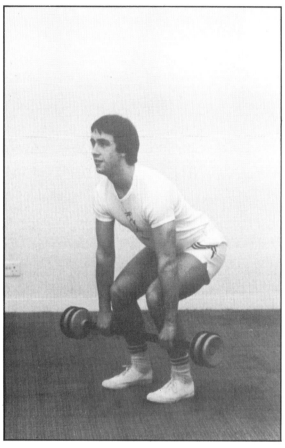

26a

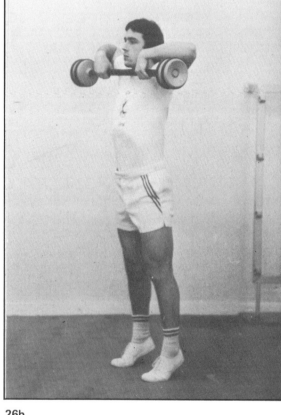

26b

Starting position: Feet hip-width apart, and insteps under the barbell. Knees bent, back flat but not vertical. Eyes front, hands in overgrasp (*26a*).

Action: Lift the barbell in a straight line to chin level. Bend the elbows to the sides as the barbell passes the top of the thighs. Come high on the toes as the barbell reaches the chest and the legs and body extend (*26b*). Lower the barbell back to the starting position and repeat.

Repetitions: Initially 10, then progress to 30-40.

Breathing: Inhale as you raise the barbell, exhale as you lower it.

2 Two–handed barbell curls

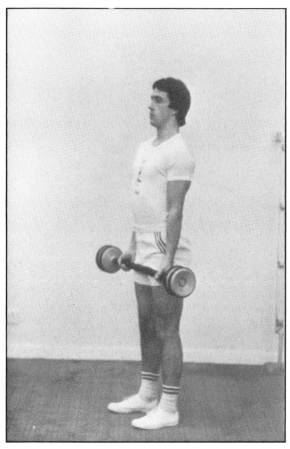

27a

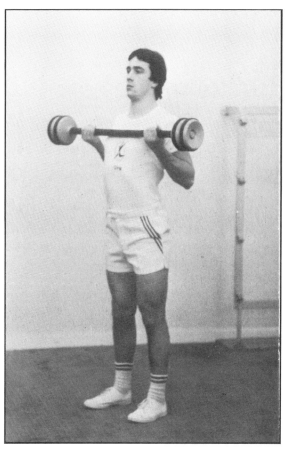

27b

Starting position: Feet hip-width apart, body erect, arms hanging by the sides. Look ahead and grip the barbell in undergrasp (*27a*).

Action: Lift the barbell in a straight line from its resting position against the thighs. As the arms bend, the elbows should be pulled backwards and close in to the chest (*27b*). Return the barbell from the end position against the chest and repeat.

Repetitions: 10 or 12 and no more.

Breathing: Inhale as you raise the barbell, exhale as you lower it.

Comments: During the exercise concentrate on a good position for head and spine. Always reach high with the head to keep the kinks out of the spine.

3 Press behind neck

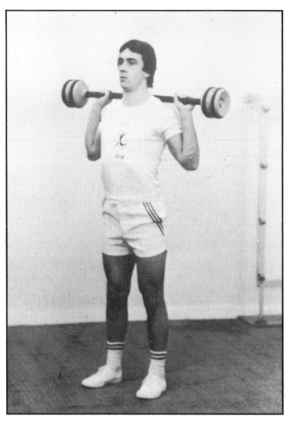

28a

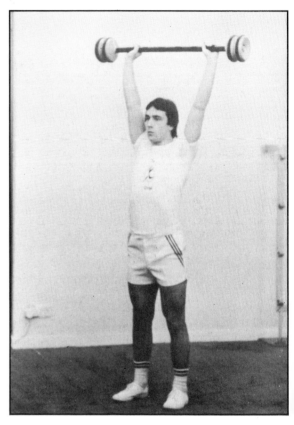

28b

Starting position: Feet hip-width apart, body erect, arms hanging by the sides. Grip the bar in overgrasp and look straight ahead (*28a*).

Action: Lift the barbell from its resting position behind the neck by extending the arms until the bar is vertically at arms' length above the head (*28b*). Return to the starting position and repeat.

Repetitions: 10 or 12 and no more.

Breathing: Inhale as you raise the barbell, exhale as you lower it. Keep a good posture throughout. Do not arch the spine.

4 Rowing exercise with barbell

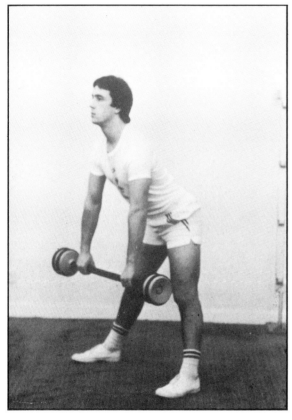

29a

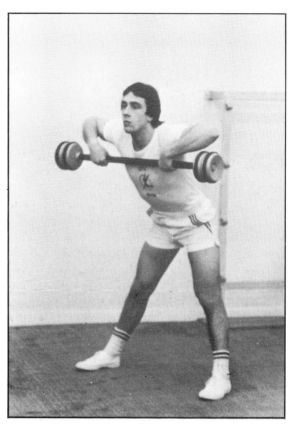

29b

Starting position: Feet hip-width apart, stand with the body erect. Grip the bar in overgrasp. Now place the feet in wide astride position and tilt the trunk to an angle of 45 degrees. The arms should hang loosely downwards, straight but relaxed (*29a*).

Action: Lift the barbell in a straight line until it touches the top of the chest. As the elbows bend, they should point sideways. The trunk should remain at 45 degrees throughout the movement (*29b*). Return to starting position and repeat.

Repetitions: 10 or 12 and no more.

Breathing: Inhale as you raise the bar, exhale as you lower it.

5 Side-to-side bends with one dumb-bell*

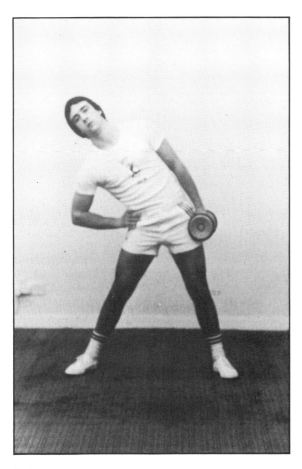

30a

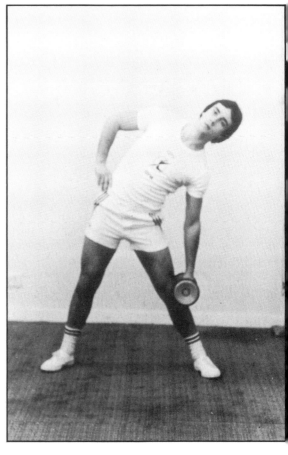

30b

Starting position: Feet very wide apart, dumb-bell held in the left hand. Arms should be straight but not tense, right hand on hip. Body should be erect, eyes looking straight ahead.

Action: Lift the dumb-bell by bending the trunk to the right side away from the dumb-bell. The arm is not involved in the exercise and should remain relaxed (*30a*). Bend as far to each side as possible, but without strain (*30b*). Pass through the erect position after every bend without stopping.

Repetitions: Start with 10 and work up to 20 or 30. Do all your repetitions on one side and then change the dumb-bell to the other side. Do not alternate from side to side.

Breathing: Breathe freely throughout.

Comments: There is a great tendency to lean forwards with the trunk. Avoid this.

6 Squat (half-knee bend) with barbell*

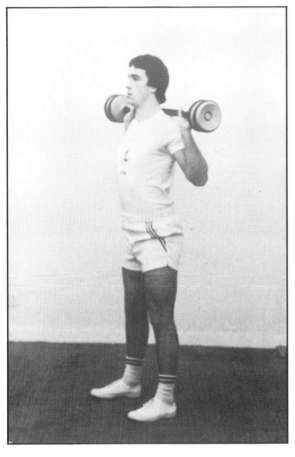

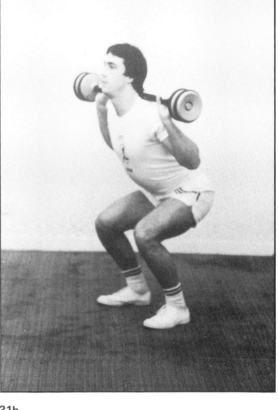

31a

31b

Starting position: Feet hip-width apart, bar held on the shoulders behind the neck in overgrasp. Hands shoulder-width apart, arms relaxed (*31a*).

Action: Lower the barbell by bending both knees. Press the hips backwards to prevent the heels from leaving the floor. The spine should be in a good postural position. It is natural for the trunk to tilt forwards as the knees bend (*31b*). *Do not go past the horizontal with the thighs.* Return to start and repeat.

Repetitions: 10 initially, and work up to 30 or 40.

Breathing: Inhale as you bend the knees, exhale as you raise the body.

Note: Following this exercise you have a choice between the press on back on floor if you do not have a bench, and the bench press proper.

7 Press on floor, or on bench, with barbell

Starting position: *On floor:* Lie on the back with barbell across chest. Hold the bar in overgrasp, hands shoulder-width apart, elbows fully bent and pointing towards the feet (*32a*).
On bench: As above, but the knees are bent as well as the elbows. The elbows should point towards the floor. The bench should be at least 1 foot high, and 3 by 1 feet in length and width respectively (*32b*).

Action: Press (lift) the bar vertically above the chest (*32c and d*). Lower and repeat. The action is the same for the floor as for the bench exercise.

Repetitions: 10 or 12 and no more.

Breathing: Inhale as you raise the bar, exhale as you lower it.

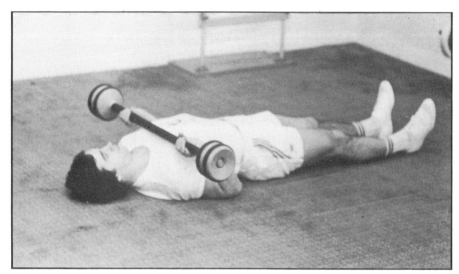

32a

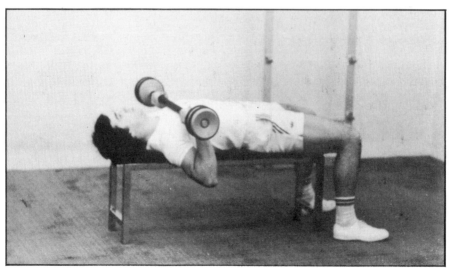

32b

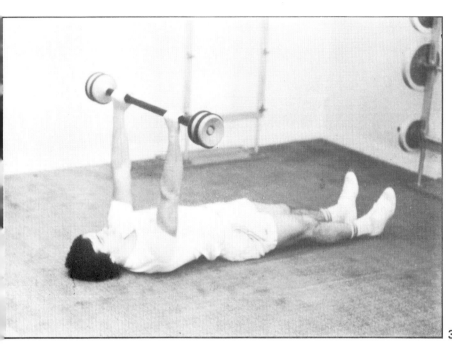

32c

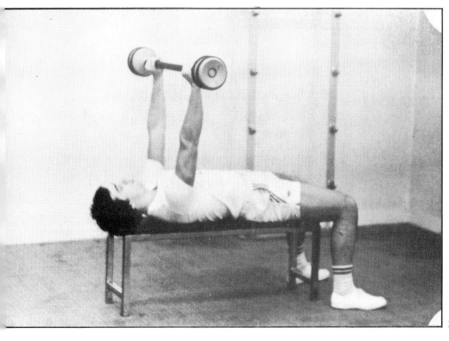

32d

8 Power cleans with barbell*

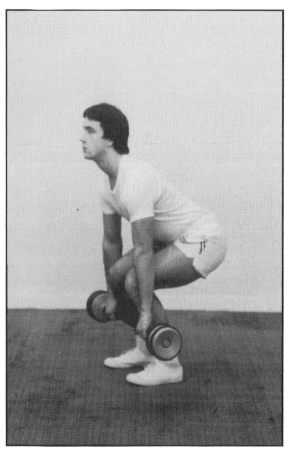

33a

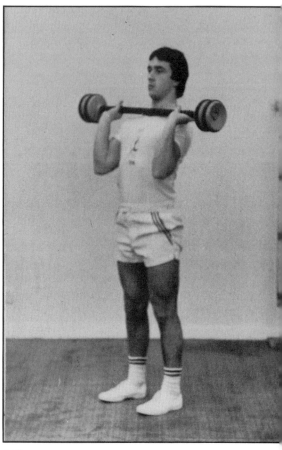

33b

Starting position: Feet hip-width apart, insteps under the bar, knees bent to 90 degrees. The back should be flat, not vertical. Grip the bar in overgrasp, look straight ahead (*33a*).

Action: Lift the bar in a straight line from the floor until it rests high on the chest. As the bar is raised, the elbows should point sideways. As the bar reaches the chest the elbows now point directly forwards. Keep a good postural spine throughout (*33b*).

Repetitons: 10 initially, then work up to 30 or 40.

Breathing: Inhale as you raise the bar, exhale as you lower it.

9 V sit-ups*

Starting position: Arms outstretched above the head whilst back lying (an inclined bench can be used for further progressions) or lie on the floor (*34a*).

Action: Raise the body into a V position and attempt to grasp the ankles (*34b*).

Repetitions: Do two groups of 10 repetitions initially. The eventual aim is two groups of 20 repetitons.

Breathing: Exhale as the trunk and legs are raised, and inhale as they are lowered.

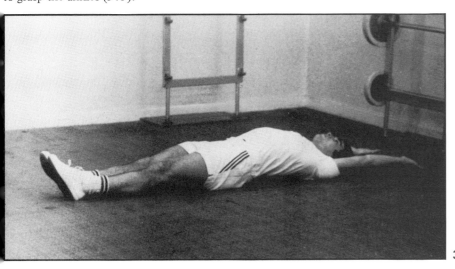

34a

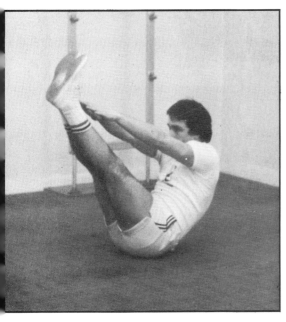

34b

10 Straight arm pull-over with barbell

(This can be performed on the floor or on a bench.)

Starting position: If lying with the back on the floor keep the legs straight. If on a bench bend the knees. Rest the bar on the thighs. Grip in overgrasp with hands shoulder-width apart (*35a and b*).

Action: Lift the bar in as large a half-circle as possible from the thighs to a horizontal arm position behind the head. Keep the arms straight, but not tense throughout the movement. Do not arch the back or overstrain the shoulder joint (*35c and d*).

Repetitions: 10 or 12 and no more.

Breathing: Inhale as you raise the barbell, and exhale as you lower it.

Comment: At the end of each repetition rest the bar momentarily on the thighs to take the tension out of the shoulder muscles. This exercise can be performed while you lie on a bench. The advantage of a bench is that you can gradually increase the range of movement in the shoulder girdle, and hence improve your mobility in that joint.

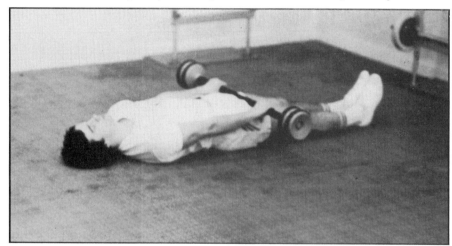

35a

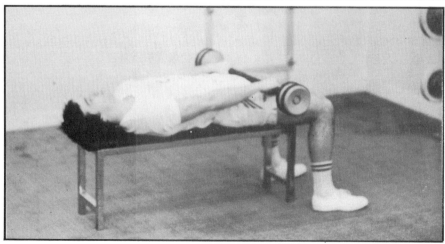

35b

Note: It is not possible to prescribe exact numbers of repetitions. When 10 or 12 repetitions are advised we suggest for the first few weeks you do no more than 10 repetitions, as you become fitter you can progress to 12. The same applies when, on the asterisked exercises, we recommend eventually 30 or 40 repetitions, the final number you do depends upon your age, state of fitness and sex.

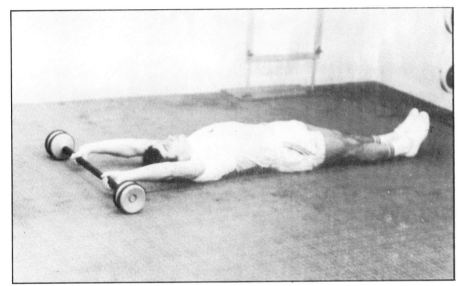

35c

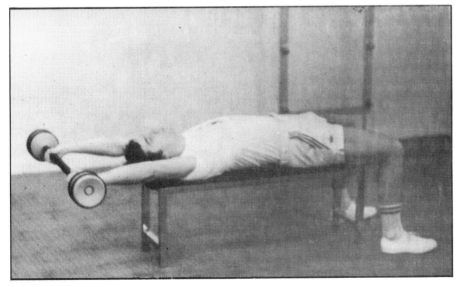

35d

Important reminder

It is important that when you return to the starting position between each repetition you relax the body as much as possible to facilitate the flow of blood. Remember, we are avoiding isometric contractions which have a deleterious effect on the circulatory system. Our rule is contraction-relaxation, contraction-relaxation. We are not concerned with maximal performance as is an Olympic athlete.

Throughout the whole schedule we are controlling what we do by careful pulse measurements, and by work loading. It is a fact that in the early stages of training, when you are only doing 10 repetitions of the exercises marked by an asterisk, you will find that your pulse rate is not being raised by very much. Once your technique has improved and you are doing higher work loads, you will find that your pulse rate approaches something near the mean you are wishing to attain. And, of course, the calculated pulse rate can never be adhered to a single beat. Below are recommended maximum and minimum mean pulse rates. You will see, for example, that a person between the ages of twenty and twenty-four years has a minimum of 130 beats per minute recommended and a maximum of 155. If he is twenty-three years of age, according to our previous calculation his work rate should be 200 − (23 + 40) = 137. This is 7 beats above his recommended *minimum mean*, and 18 beats below his recommended *maximum mean*. The final figure depends upon all the other factors we have previously discussed. If the twenty-three year old has over the weeks eliminated his handicap of 40, his maximum rate would be 200 − (23 + 177) beats per minute. You will see that this is 30 beats higher than the recommended maximum mean pulse rate − it is, but the mean rate does not mean the maximum rate. If his mean was 177 beats per minute it would also be his maximum, and such a system of working would make nonsense of our physiological sequence, and would be harmful for our exerciser.

Fig. 12 Recommended minimum and maximum pulse rates

| Ages | Mean pulse | |
	Minimum	Maximum
20-24	130	155
25-29	128	150
30-34	125	145
35-39	120	142
40-44	118	138
45-49	116	136
50-54	114	125
55-60	110	118
60+	105	115

Note: If you are exceeding your *mean* pulse rate during the schedule, then you must reduce your work load. Remember we are concerned with protective, not competitive exercise, and that our figures are based on measuring hundreds of test volunteers.

Fig. 13 Recommended minimum and maximum repounds per minute

| Ages | Repounds per minute | |
	Minimum	Maximum
20-24	4000	6000
25-29	4500	6500
30-34	4500	6500
35-39	4000	6000
40-44	3500	5500
45-49	3000	5000
50-54	2500	4500
55-60	2000	4000
60+	1750	3000

Note: This chart should be used in conjunction with fig. 12.

An example of how the repounds per minute is calculated

Exercise	Pounds	Repetitions
1 High chin pull	20	30
2 Curls	20	12
3 Press behind neck	20	12
4 Rowing	20	12
5 Side bends	15	40
6 Squat	20	30
7 Bench press	20	12
8 Power clean	20	30
9 V sit-ups	15	20
		(Eventually 2 sets of 20)
10 Pull-over	10	12
	180 lb x	210 reps.

Time taken: 16 minutes

Repounds per minutes = $\dfrac{180 \times 210}{16}$ = 2363 repounds per minute

Note: This calculation is only relevant when you are working at the maximum number of repetitions for the large muscle group exercises.

Summary

By now you will be armed with a vast amount of theoretical detail, the better to enable you to derive the greatest benefit from the practical work. Before we tell you how to apply the schedule to your own use, we feel it will benefit you if we summarize what we have said about the apparatus schedule and its theoretical foundation.

1 We assume you have completed at least the first two non-apparatus schedules. It is better to have done all four, but you must have done at least two if you are a man. The ladies may not wish to use weights at all — though very many do, and the adaptations for them are on pages 113-14. Certainly the ladies will find the fourth non-apparatus schedule very tough, and can do themselves as much good by concentrating on the first three.

2 You know how to take your pulse and you know why you take it.

3 You know that the work loading system uniquely designed and tested works in conjunction with pulse rate control to assist in the accurate charting of your progress.

4 You know that our aim is stamina, as well as strength and suppleness, and that this stamina training depends on doing the exercises without pause at an even tempo.

5 You know how to calculate your pulse rate and that in the early stages you are only concerned with the maximum pulse rate recommended according to the calculations. And because the maximum pulse rate is going to refer to the exercises marked by an asterisk you need only take your pulse rate after those exercises.

6 You know in great detail that the key factors in the apparatus schedule refer to pulse rate means and repounds per minute. *What we have not yet said is that these mean weights and mean pulse rates* shown in figs. 12 and 13 *are only relevant when you decide to test your progress.* In the section entitled 'The Test Day' (see pages 112-13) — we explain just how you use the charts.

7 You know, if you have read the book carefully, that we are concerned with a safe programme, and that our aim is protective exercise. We cannot too strongly emphasize that the objective in the weight training programme is not to get to the maximum number of repetitions as soon as possible. Do not work too quickly. Always work according to your heart rate as indicated by pulse measurements. Do not forget our warning about the potential dangers of near maximal isometric contraction.

Your weight training programme in action

You are now ready to begin the apparatus schedule. The following precedure is recommended.

1 Do the five mobility exercises in the usual way.
2 Take a weight of 10 lb and use this weight throughout to begin with.
3 Start with Exercise 1, the high chin pull and do 12 repetitions.
4 Go on to Exercise 2, the curls, without a pause, and do 10 repetitions.
5 Continue through the whole schedule doing 12 repetitions for the exercises marked *, and 10 repetitions for all the other exercises. *You will never do more than* 10 repetitions for these exercises.
6 Take your pulse after Exercises 5 and 9. We suggest 5 and 9 because the first is half-way through the schedule and, according to the physiological sequence, you should be approaching your maximum, and after Exercise 9 you should be at your maximum or thereabouts. These are both large muscle group exercises. There is nothing to prevent you taking your pulse after all the asterisked exercises, but the more often you stop to take your pulse, the less cardio-vascular effect is the schedule having. In any case, always take your pulse rate if you feel you are working too hard.
7 *Three golden rules.* If when your are working through the schedule,
   a. The tempo at which you do each repetition of a certain exercise slows down
   b. You cannot work without rest periods
   c. You exceed your maximum pulse rate
   then you must reduce the weight your are using.
8 If, on the other hand,
   a. You are doing the repetitions at a brisk constant tempo
   b. You are nowhere near your maximum pulse rate on the exercises marked *
   c. You are completing the schedule in less than 12 minutes
   then you must increase the resistance by adding more weight. Never increase the number of repetitions beyond the maximum of 40 on the asterisked exercises and 10 on all the others.
9 Once you feel comfortable with 12 and 10 repetitions and you are fulfilling all other requirements, then gradually increase the number of repetitions on the asterisked exercises. Increase them by four or five a session over two or three weeks. Once you are doing 30-40 repetitions on the asterisked

exercises, and you are obeying the three golden rules, then it is time for you to increase the poundage.
10 *Increasing the resistance.* It would be impossible, not to say useless, to prescribe specific weights for you to use. Your guidelines for safe and efficient working reside in the application of pulse rate control. When you come to increase the weights you are using you must experiment. If you started with 10 pounds on each exercise then see what happens when you add 2 more pounds. Then, with this higher work load, go back to doing 10 repetitions of the non-asterisked exercises and 12 of all the others.
11 Work up to 30-40 repetitions on the asterisked exercises as before.
12 Once you can do the new schedule at the same tempo, without pause and without increasing your recommended pulse rate you are ready to progress again.
13 Make sure the increases in weight are slight.
14 If you find that your pulse rate is higher than it should be check to see that you are not doing the exercises at too great a tempo.

The test day

After several weeks' work during which time you have been perfecting your lifting techniques and accustoming yourself to taking your pulse rate after the large muscle group exercises, the time comes when mean pulse rates and mean work loads are of great significance.

Let us suggest a hypothetical situation. Here is a man of thirty who, by doing the non-apparatus schedule, has succeeded in eliminating his handicap and is working at a recommended maximum pulse rate of 200-30 beats per minutes. His maximum is 170 beats per minute, and that after the maximum of 40 repetitions on Exercise 5 and Exercise 9 he took his pulse rate and found it about right. We say 'about right', because after Exercise 9 it was considerably higher than 170 beats, but after Exercise 5 it was noticeably lower. He was working without pause and at the same even tempo throughout the schedule. He now needs a more accurate guide to his actual work. This is what he does.

Test day 1

1 He has his chart showing the ten exercises and beside each exercise he has a column in which he can write the poundage he is using, the number of repetitions he is doing and his pulse rate.
2 He works through the whole schedule noting the number of repetitions and the weight he is using.

3 He takes the time from the start to the finish of the schedule *excluding* the mobility exercises.

4 He now calculates his repounds per minute.

Test day 2

1 He duplicates the exact conditions for the Day 1 test and works through the schedule again. Particular care is taken to see that the tempo is the same as it was on Day 1.

2 After Exercise 3, the press behind neck, he takes his pulse.

3 After Exercise 8, the power clean, he takes his pulse rate.

4 At the end of the schedule he adds the two rates together and finds a mean pulse rate, i.e. he adds the two pulse rates together and divides them by two. Let us assume that after the first exercise his pulse was 130 and after the second it was 170. The mean is 300 divided by two = 150. If we turn to fig. 12 we will see that he is working at a slightly higher mean than we recommended, so he should reduce the resistance slightly. If we look at his repounds per minutes we may see that he is working at over 7000 repounds per minutes and that this is in excess of our maximum. Our pulse test is confirmed by our work loading calculation.

A final word

The above test is only to be done when you have been working at the schedule for two or three months, and only after you have achieved maximum repetitions with the asterisked exercises.

As with all recommended means they cannot be regarded as the last word. Some of you may well be working at over 10,000 repounds per minute and with pulse rates considerably higher than our recommended means. This probably means that you are moving out of the realms of protective fitness and into those of competitive fitness. If that is the case, excellent. But for many of you our norms will suffice to give you the protection you need. Do not attempt to speed up your progress artificially. We are concerned with protection and in some cases rehabilitation. As we have explained, the physiological sequence of peaks and troughs will mean that at the peak of the schedule you will be exceeding your calculated maximum pulse rate, and that at the lowest trough you will be working below your recommended maximum. A *mean* pulse rate is not a *maximum* pulse rate. The peaks are designed to increase the work load on the heart, the troughs are designed to give you relative rests so that you can continue the schedule without pause.

The important thing is that you work for about 20 minutes three times a week and that you obey the three golden rules. By the time you are doing maximum repetitions on the asterisked exercises you will know whether or not you are overdoing it. You will be able to interpret the activity of your heart just by 'feeling' its beat. Don't be confused by what was said earlier on the difficulty of deducing anything accurate by empirical observation. We are now talking about your own experience of your own heart under your own control. That is very different from watching somebody else for the first time and making deductions. Let pulse rate control be your servant, not your master.

Weight training for ladies

Ladies who wish to embark on the apparatus schedule, and it is hoped many will, have a slightly modified programme. They do all the exercises the men do except two. For Exercise 2, the curls, the ladies do vertical rowing, and instead of Exercise 6, the squat, they do squats on toes. Women should work with 10 lb throughout, and they should reduce their pulse rate means by 10 per cent.

Weight training equipment

Here is some advice on how best you can equip yourself to do weight training. Ideally, of course, your aim on the exercise programme is to be able to graduate to the use of weights. Only then can you gain full benefit from The Murray Work Loading System. You probably realize by now that weights do range from a few ounces to several hundred-weight, and that you can do valuable work using very light weights.

Barbells are 1 inch steel bars or tubes varying in length from 4 to 6 or 7 feet to which metal discs are attached at each end. Dumb-bells are short versions of barbells, about 1-foot long, to which again, adjustable weights are attached. Barbells are used for two-handed exercises, and dumb-bells for single-handed exercises where the arms are being exercised independently of the rest of the body. The discs attached to the bars can weigh anything from a few ounces – or even less – to almost anything one requires.

Because weight training as discussed here is for protective health and fitness, not for competition, the bar or tubes we use need not be longer than 4 feet. The discs on the dumb-bells and barbells are of the smaller size, and are slipped onto the end of the bar and attached by means of a collar. There is a sleeve into which the bars are inserted which

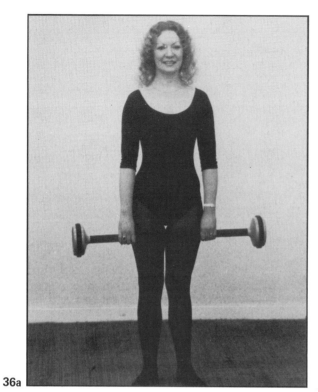

36a

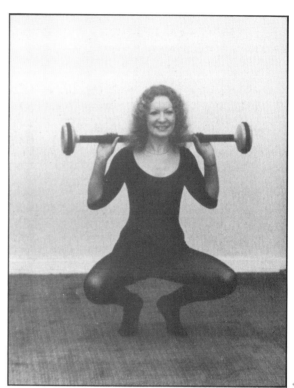

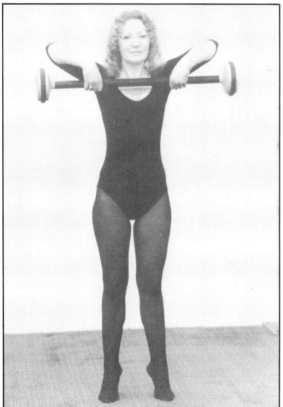

36b

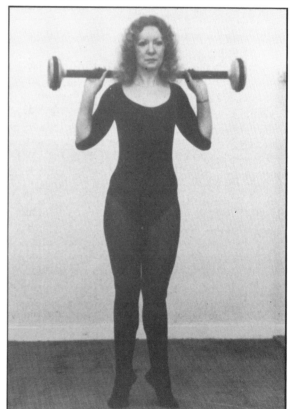

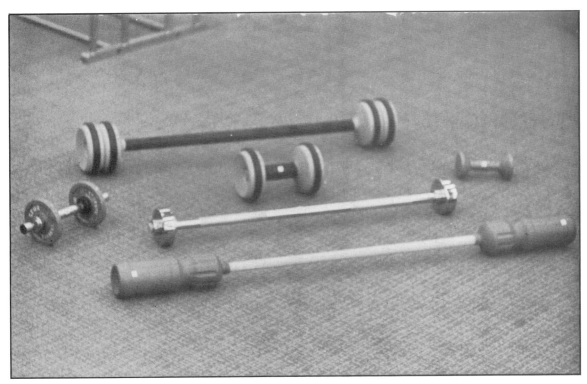

38 Weight training equipment: *rear,* special adjustable plastic barbell and dumb-bell (*centre*); *centre left,* disc loading dumb-bell; *centre right,* solid dumb-bell; *centre,* chromium-plated disc loading barbell; *and front,* home-made barbell using broomstick and plastic bottles.

prevents the discs from coming inwards. The sleeve also enables you to use a revolving grip in safety and comfort. The equipment used in some of the exercises in the book is of another variety. The discs are hollow and of a heavy duty plastic. They can be filled to the weight required with either water or sand. These new types of discs, which are made by Jungeling Limited, are adequate for our type of fitness training.

If at this stage you are concerned with cost, then you should begin with home-made weights which, perhaps not quite as comfortable and safe to use, are adequate for your early training. However, the cost of a set of weights is not prohibitive. Indeed, when set against possible loss of earnings, not to say loss of health, the value is incalculably good!

For home-made weights in the early stages excellent results can be obtained by filling the normal plastic bottle, such as some types of washing-up liquid bottles, with sand and water. The weight will, of course, depend on the size of the bottle and how much you fill it. This means that when you see two-handed barbell exercises shown in the book, you will have to adapt your home-made weight's use. You will do the exercises with your home-made dumb-bell in each hand. It is possible to make a barbell by filling two plastic bottles with sand and wedging them onto each end of a broomstick.

However, in the long term, once you have convinced yourself of the benefits of weight training, there is no doubt that you should invest in proper equipment. It is safer, it will last you more than a lifetime, and can be accurately adjusted to suit your changing requirements — and can be used by all members of your family.

Postscript

The BBC fitness project

Over a period of sixteen years Al Murray at the City Gymnasium had proved a thousand times over the value and benefits to be gained from using a safe, progressive, pulse-controlled method of exercising fit and unfit adults in the three main areas of mobility, strength and stamina. Each is vital, for without any one of these factors, daily life loses something of its vigour and enjoyment. You need only look at the medical records and watch or talk to the members young and old, about how they felt, even after only two or three months, to know that the methods are totally successful.

The big problem was, 'How could more people benefit from the system or was it only to be limited to the lucky few? Even with Al Murray's energy and enthusiasm, one man alone with his small staff of Margarethe Holfeld and Frank Shipman could not hope to spread the gospel. What was needed was help — someone who could see the value of the work and who was in a position to back him and help spread the work — in fact, a 'fairy godmother'.

In 1976 such a person appeared in the form of Brigit Barry, a producer with the BBC. During his involvement on interview, Al had the chance to talk to Brigit about his work and invited her to visit the Gym to see for herself. Brigit was producing The 60-70-80 Show, a television series for the retired. The programmes, which aimed to cover every aspect of pre- and post-retirement, had started in 1975. During the first year Brigit had been very struck by the tremendous variations in physical fitness amongst the retired people she met; she was interested to find out, on their behalf, whether it was practically possible at retirement age to do anything positive about improving fitness. Brigit was considering the possibility of The 60-70-80 Show acting as catalyst for a research project into fitness in retired people.

It only took a short time at the City Gym to convince Brigit that the method used there might form the basis for such a research project and she at once set her mind to planning the way in which such a television-based research project could be presented. The result of her ingenuity and organization was a group of twenty volunteers who would follow the 60-70-80 fitness project for 12 weeks taught by Jackie Billis who was specifically trained by Al at the City Gym for the job. Perhaps the most exciting aspect was the involvement of Malcolm Carruthers and his team who carried out a series of medical tests at intervals during the project, to produce scientific evidence as to the physiological improvements brought about in the body by the exercise programme. The cost of this was covered by the British Heart Foundation.

Thus, from January to March 1976 the 60-70-80 fitness project ran twice a week with medical tests and filming taking place at the start, the halfway mark and at the end. The results were even better than Al and Malcolm had hoped for and when the final programme was filmed Malcolm was able to show the improvements which had occurred, i.e. lower pulse, blood pressure, cholesterol and coagulants. In addition, the volunteers themselves showed and explained how much better they felt as a result of their 12 weeks of exercise. There was little doubt as to the success of the project but the series ended and it could well have been the end of a happy brief encounter with more people aware of what they could and should do to keep fit and well, but with no one to help and advise.

Fortunately for Al, Brigit although permanently under the pressure of ongoing and new work with the BBC, was not prepared to let the case rest. She was determined that what had been proved should not be lost. As a result of her drive and enthusiasm, she persuaded the British Heart Foundation and the Inner London Education Authority to sponsor the training of three full-time Adult Education physical education lecturers at the City Gymnasium with Al Murray. The aim was to spread his expertise and understanding into adult evening classes where the general public could find a suitable and safe way of exercising.

During the six months' part-time training, Graham Jones, Brian Holding and Philippa Davenport were put through the mill. All three had physical education teaching qualifications and considerable experience in the field, plus a background of anatomy and physiology which was essential for the understanding of the unfit adult. Was it enough? Systematically they realized how little they did know in certain vital areas and then slowly and steadily they rebuilt their knowledge and confidence to use the practical and theoretical side of the work to the best advantage.

It was not enough to demonstrate the exercises properly or to notice and correct the faults. They had to understand why and be able to explain to the members and later to their own students the reasons for the exercises being done in a certain way and in a certain order and the effect that each one has on the body. It was necessary to understand the factors contributing to coronary heart disease — the biggest killer of our time — and to pick up early symptoms of possible trouble through pulse checks and discussions about each individual's lifestyle. In addition they needed to know the safe progressions of repetitions, speed and weights to be used and above all to know how to adapt the exercises for those with joint or muscle conditions which prevented them carrying out the normal schedule.

Working as trainees at the City Gym was no picnic but the help and encouragement given by Al, Margarethe and Frank helped to give confidence and conviction as to the value of the work in hand and after six months the first chances came to set up adult classes entitled Fitness for the Over 40s.

At both Eltham and Lansbury Institutes the classes progressed from small pilot projects to popular and well-accepted units of the PE provision for adults. These classes fill a most valuable gap for those who wanted to follow some form of active leisure after several years of inactivity and who felt they would not be able to cope with the regular ladies' keep fit or men's fitness classes.

At the same time the ripples from Brigit's 'pebble in the pond' were spreading still wider as the Health Education Council decided to run a pilot tutors' course as part of their 'Look After Yourself' campaign again using Al's ideas for the exercises in their booklet. Philippa Davenport was asked to teach the practical area of what was now seen as a three-sided course comprising practical, theory and relaxation. As a result, in the summer of 1978, tutors from London and the Home Counties were chosen from hundreds of applicants to attend and complete the course. They came from a wide range of backgrounds, including health education, adult education and further and higher education establishments. They were thus able to spread their knowledge to groups in all these fields.

In the spring of 1979, the ILEA kept the circles widening by inviting Philippa Davenport and Graham Jones to run a course specially for adult education tutors and invited applications from all the institutes. From sixteen applicants, ten finally qualified as panel tutors for 'Look After Yourself – Fitness for the Over 40s' and more classes appeared in institute prospectuses to which locals could go at a relatively small charge.

At this point Graham left London to take up a post in Cambridge and when the call for a follow-up project for 60-70-80 came from the BBC it was up to Philippa to provide the staff for what was to be a much larger medical survey than the original group of twenty.

A meeting in the autumn of 1978 of the Greater London Pre-Retirement Council brought many offers, from industry, commerce and health areas, of groups of volunteers for a new fitness project. After 12 months of fund raising, preparation of tutors, medical arrangements and questionnaires, September 1979 saw the project launched by a filming day in the Blue Peter garden and eleven groups started a 12-week exercise programme carefully laid down by Philippa to ensure that conditions were as similar as possible for each group. Equipment was discussed and shown to the groups before the project started, with the emphasis on the fact that a home-made bar and weights were quite adequate and many volunteers subsequently produced their own. By visiting and encouraging, Philippa was able to check the groups' progress and the results of the project confirmed the early encouraging findings. When the project finished several groups were loth to give up and made requests for their tutors to continue. At the same time, health education units were requesting a course for their own staff to be trained in the Al Murray methods.

The ILEA have a further tutors' course arranged for spring 1980 to be taught by Philippa Davenport with twenty-five aiming to qualify and it is hoped that the Health Education Council too will run a further course. It is essential that the thousands of middle-aged and older adults who are being encouraged to improve their level of fitness, in order to enjoy life to the full, should be able to do so in the safe and competent hands of well-trained staff who understand the problems and additional care which is needed for this very large group of our present population.

Let us hope that the expertise and hard work continue to spread so that the whole country can benefit from a fitter and happier old age.

'Fitness may not add years to life but it adds life to years'.

Report on BBC 60-70-80 Show study of exercise in people of retirement age by

M.E. Carruthers, MD, MRC Path., MRCGP, Director of Clinical Laboratories, Maudsley and Bethlem Royal Hospitals

The number of people completing the study was 185, of whom 163 were in the exercising group and the remainder in an important control group for comparison. Detailed medical tests were carried out before and after the three months' exercise programme. The study showed a wide range of benefits even with the limited amount of exercise which, as in the previous smaller pilot study, gave the impression that the participants were becoming medically fitter and seemingly younger week by week.

This increasing fitness was seen most clearly in the heart and circulation where the studies at the end of the exercise showed that on average the heart was beating more slowly and efficiently and the blood pressure had come down. The number of red blood corpuscles, their volume, and the amount of the oxygen-carrying pigment haemoglobin, had also all increased encouragingly. There was also good news on the chemical front with reduction of all three of the main important types of fat in the blood, including the dreaded cholesterol. Calcium levels had also decreased slightly, and an enzyme which is concerned with bone building had increased, suggesting that a strengthening activity in the bone had occurred.

Questionnaires concentrating on mood, drive and anxiety levels were regarded as a most important part of the project, since it was felt objectively that exercise improved morale and increased *joie de vivre* in the elderly. The results confirmed these beliefs and gave some of the first evidence obtained in this country that increased mental fitness goes hand in hand with increased physical fitness, a most important factor in adding life to years rather than just years to life.

The exercising volunteers met once each week for a training session and practised the exercises at home as well as following a walking programme. The fact that there were no real accidents, injuries or unpleasant side effects experienced by any people on the exercise programme, and that nearly all completed it, is good evidence of the basis of safe and interesting exercises designed by Al Murray and described in our Sports Council paperback *F/40 (Fitness on 40 minutes a week)*. This method was an abridged version of Al Murray's comprehensive method as used at the City Gym which follows the principle that mental training should be encouraged as much as physical training in keeping the elderly active. Meditation can be considered exercise of the mind and can produce a new and positive approach to life and tranquility without tranquillizers, and sleep without pills. A simple form of Western meditation is Autogenics described elsewhere in this book or taught in greater depth by the Autogenic Training Centre in London.

The success of this project is a great tribute to the training, enthusiasm and teaching abilities of all the instructors on the programme. We have already seen signs that this enthusiasm is contagious and other Civil Servants and industrial groups of people about retirement age are already starting to form groups of their own.

The principle of exercise used throughout the project was that it should be SAFE.

S *(Safety)* – This was ensured both by the dynamic rather than static form of exercises carried out, and by attention to pulse rate and perceived exertion.

A *(Acceptability)* – The exercise programme was varied and the group setting provided a great deal of encouragement.

F *(Fitness producing)* – The volunteers felt the benefits of the programme for themselves quite early on and could see that they were getting stronger and more supple as well as taking part in the mental and physical checks.

E *(Economy)*– This was in terms of time in that the exercise programme took only half an hour, two or three times a week, and in terms of space a large number of people could exercise in a small area and did not need expensive equipment.

Further results of the study are still being analysed by computer but initially there seems to be a wide range of benefits to the exercise volunteers.

Index